Residential and Boarding Education and Care for Young People: A Model for Good Practice

In the UK alone some 140,000 young people live away from home in a wide range of residential, boarding and custodial establishments. Care of these children and young people has been subject to much recent legislation about quality of care and child protection issues, as well as a drive towards evidence-based standards.

This innovative book identifies the key elements of good management and practice common to all residential child care settings, whether hospital unit, boarding school, children's home, special school or custodial care establishment. The author outlines a model developed under the auspices of the Joseph Rowntree Foundation and based on over 35 years experience in practice and research in over 500 residential settings. The main components of the model are:

- the environment
- the legal framework
- developmental issues
- time-related issues.

In each case the key factors for practice and management are discussed and key roles and outcomes identified.

This book is invaluable reading for anyone working with children and young people in all forms of residential and boarding education and care, and for students of childcare at undergraduate and post-qualifying levels, in the UK and internationally. The framework can be readily applied to training, assessment of standards, inspections, and research and development.

Ewan Anderson is Emeritus Professor at the University of Durham and Honorary Professor in the Social Work and Development Unit, University of York, where he works on residential and boarding education and care. He holds doctorates in geography, politics and residential education and has published fourteen books. He is a former president of the International Federation of Educative Communities (England and Wales branch) and a member of four national standards committees.

Residential and Boarding Education and Care for Young People: A Model for Good Practice

Ewan W Anderson

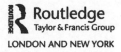

Routledge
Taylor & Francis Group

LONDON AND NEW YORK

First published in 2005 by Routledge
2 Park Square, Milton Park, Abingdon,
Oxfordshire, OX14 4RN
Tel: +44 020 7017 6000
Fax: +44 020 7017 6699

Simultaneously published in the USA and Canada
by Taylor & Francis Inc
711 Third Avenue, New York, NY 10017

Routledge is an imprint of the Taylor & Francis Group

Transferred to Digital Printing 2005

Typeset in Sabon MT by J&L Composition, Filey, North Yorkshire

British Library Cataloguing in Publication Data
A catalogue record for this book is available from the British
Library

Library of Congress Cataloging in Publication Data
A catalogue record has been requested

ISBN 0–415–30554–3 (hbk)
ISBN 0–415–30555–1 (pbk)

To Rosie Baillon, with whom I have worked for the past ten years, for all her application, diligence and constructive ideas but above all for her friendship and support.

Contents

Figures

Preface

For a variety of reasons some young people, for at least part of their lives, live away from their families in residential and boarding education and care communities. The balance between education: formal and informal, and care: social, health and custodial, differs from community to community but all are living and learning environments. Although they may be labelled as schools, colleges, homes, units, centres or institutions, all have a focus upon residential or boarding education, the informal learning which occurs when groups of young people and dedicated staff work together and share the daily activities of life.

How this concept of residential or boarding education has been developed in the various settings has remained a constant fascination for me during more than thirty-five years of practice and research. During that time, it has been my privilege and pleasure to share the normal activities of living in more than five hundred establishments, predominantly in the United Kingdom (UK) but also in twenty-seven other countries covering five continents. I have also benefited greatly from the support and advice from many chairmen during my twenty-six years as research officer and boarding adviser to the Boarding Schools' Association. Apart from practice in the different settings in which I have stayed, I also ran what may be collectively described as residential units in the Royal Navy, a boarding school, a teacher training college and a university. In fact, my interest in the subject was aroused even earlier as a boarder who was able, through sport, to visit an array of schools and colleges. My horizons were later greatly broadened by three giants in the field who became close friends: Haydn Davies Jones, with whom I worked at Newcastle University; Barbara Kahan, who invited me to become a member of the Wagner Development Group; and John Gittins, an examiner for my doctoral thesis.

Given the wide range of variables, residential and boarding education and care is complex. However, from any standpoint – logical, academic or practical – it is clear that the commonalities outweigh the differences between the sectors. As a result, there is the potential for realistic transfer, not only of practice and ideas but also of staff and in some cases young people, between the sectors. It was with an emphasis upon this transfer value that the York Group, comprising practitioners and researchers from across the variety of settings, was established in 1989. I owe a particular debt of gratitude to the members of the York Group who, between them, have produced so many interesting discussions and seminars. The three York Days, research seminars with a wide participation at national level, have been extremely stimulating.

As one response to the key issues aired in all these different fora and as an attempt to produce a more formal structure for the generation of training and research, a model has been developed, for which I bear responsibility. In this context I must thank Chrysa Apps for all her encouragement, and the Joseph Rowntree Foundation for generously funding the design, trialling and production of the course for residential and boarding staff. The model was initiated during research for the course. In this book, the model has been used to identify and analyse the main facets of residential and boarding education and care. The book is aimed at practitioners, managers, trainers and researchers in the hope that it will help to stimulate some ideas for research-based practice and evidence-based research.

In writing this book, I am particularly indebted to all those practitioners who, over the years and in a variety of settings, have shared with me their thoughts on how to live and work effectively with young people living away from home in groups. I am indebted also to the many young people in all types of setting who have offered me their ideas on the issues of residence and boarding. I thank members of staff in the universities to which I have been attached and to all those who have been members of the York Group or its predecessor. I am especially grateful to my son Lewis, a diligent and compassionate social worker, for continuing guidance on the subject matter. I should also like to thank my wife Sian, who helped run the various residential units and the Department of Education and Science Clearing House for Maintained Boarding Schools, and who remains a lay inspector of homes, for improving the script, both factually and stylistically. As in much of my work, I owe particular thanks to Ian Cool who converted my ideas and rough sketches into sophisticated figures. Finally, a special debt of gratitude goes to Rosie Baillon, herself an experienced practitioner, not only for her meticulous attention to detail in typing the script but also for her informed comments and advice which have significantly improved its quality.

Ewan Anderson
Durham

Acronyms

ACPC   Area Child Protection Committee
AD/HD   attention deficit/hyperactivity disorder
BMA   British Medical Association
CAMHS   Child and Adolescent Mental Health Services
CCETSW   Central Council for Education and Training in Social Work
CRB   Criminal Records Bureau
DfE   Department for Education
DfEE   Department for Education and Employment
DfES   Department for Education and Skills
DoH   Department of Health
DTO   Detention and Training Order
EU   European Union
FE   further education
FICE   International Federation for Educative Communities
           (title in English)
HE   higher education
HIV   human immunodeficiency virus
HMP   Her Majesty's Prison
HMSO   Her Majesty's Stationery Office
LASU   Local Authority Secure Unit
LEA   Local Education Authority
LSCB   Local Safeguarding Children Board
NATSPEC   Association of National Specialist Colleges
NCB   National Children's Bureau
NHS   National Health Service
NICAPS   National In-patient Child and Adolescent Psychiatry Study
NTO   National Training Organisation
NVQ   National Vocational Qualification
PSD   personal and social development
PSHCE   personal, social, health and citizenship education
PSHE   personal, social and health education

QNIC	Quality Network for In-patient CAMHS (Child and Adolescent Mental Health Services)
RGN	Registered General Nurse
SATs	standard assessment tasks
SEN	special educational needs
SPCK	Society for the Propagation of Christian Knowledge
STC	Secure Training Centre
SVQ	Scottish Vocational Qualification
TOPSS	Training Organisation for the Personal Social Services
TSO	The Stationery Office
UK	United Kingdom
YJB	Youth Justice Board
YOI	Young Offender Institution
YOT	Youth Offending Team

Chapter 1

Introduction

The term 'residential and boarding education and care' covers all children and young people living in groups away from their families. There is a wide variation among the types of setting in which they live but they all share a living and learning environment. Their fundamental needs, concerning care, health and education, are those of all children and young people, and the residential group is distinguished by the fact that these needs are provided outside the family through group living. Foster care and adoption are, of course, also extra-familial but involve closer and more intense relationships with the adults and any group living involved is normally on a smaller scale than that found in the smallest children's home (Irving *et al.*, 1993).

Given the factors of basic needs, location and lifestyles which they share, it is not surprising that, across the field of residential and boarding education and care there are more commonalities than differences. Although the focus may be upon education, health, social care or custodial care, the aims and the means by which these are achieved are largely common. The purpose of this book is to discuss the development and application of a generic model which encapsulates these commonalities and identifies the significant distinctions. In continental Europe the term 'social pedagogue' is used for the member of the residential staff who in all the required ways supports the children and young people while living with them. Good practice for the social pedagogue across all the types of setting is similar, the differences being more of emphasis rather than activity. Using the model, the core components of generic good practice are identified and described and the key discussion points are addressed. The model itself has been constructed over many years of action research across the field, of discussions with practitioners, researchers and administrators and of time spent talking to the children and young people (O'Quigley, 2000). Many of the ideas were brought together initially as a result of the *Children Act* (1989) and research on its implementation for the Department of Health (DoH).

The *Children Act* (1989) extends consideration of children and young people from those solely looked after by local authorities in children's homes, and rationalises the legal framework for safeguarding the welfare of children and young people living away from home in institutions such as private and voluntary homes, independent and maintained schools, and private and National Health Service (NHS) hospitals (DoH, 1989b). Subsequently, the framework has been enhanced, partly through the *Care Standards Act* (2000), and now includes young people under the age of 18 in further education (FE) colleges and in custodial care. Therefore, all children and young people living in residence, in ex-familial settings, are covered except for those under the age of 18 in military training establishments and possibly, depending upon how the hostel is defined, those of the same age group in refugee hostels. The best estimate for the number of children and young people in residential and boarding education and care, whether or not they are included under the Act, is approximately 145,000.

Despite the two Acts and Amendments, the perception persists in government and among many authorities and agencies that residential education and care equates with children's homes. There are at present just over 7,000 children and young people in children's homes. Thus the issue of residential education and care appears to be concerned with a very small minority. In fact, the total is almost half that classified as children and young people in need, on whom the government understandably focuses maximum attention. Even if the mainstream boarding component is removed from the total, there are still approximately ten times as many children and young people in residence as there are in children's homes.

The fact that there are so many children and young people living away from home in groups in such a variety of settings requires official recognition. The different sectors of residential and boarding education and care have developed in a variety of ways but much of the good practice and indeed much of the tradition is shared. Therefore, there is the opportunity to identify common issues and problems and to examine the potential for the transfer of good practice. Indeed, the Department for Education and Skills (DfES) is currently examining the feasibility of moving children and young people from a number of other settings into mainstream boarding schools. Other such transfers between the types of setting have been successfully made. A good example is provided by a young person who moved from a Local Authority Secure Unit (LASU) to a residential special school for behaviour, emotional and social development difficulties from which he attended classes in a local maintained boarding school. He eventually moved into the boarding house of that school. Meanwhile, the staff at the two schools, almost for the first time, became aware of each other, and very fruitful staff exchanges were initiated. This is but one instance, but it does illustrate the potential for the transfer of both children or young people and staff.

Types of setting

As a result of regional meetings, visits and action research, the number of types of setting in which children and young people live away from home in groups is currently considered to be nineteen. The reason for the diffidence is that many settings cross the boundaries of the types, particularly among special schools, and the exact subdivision depends upon definition. However, the inventory has been discussed in detail at meetings with government departments, agencies, administrators, researchers and practitioners and no amendments have been forthcoming. Yet, as society changes, so new types of establishment will probably be required. At present the Youth Justice Board (YJB) is examining the possibility of developing care units intermediate between custodial care and community care. Another interesting example may be seen in Malta which presents something of a microcosm of the situation which obtains in the UK. The problems are much the same as those in the UK but the requirement, as a result of the numbers of children and young people involved and the costs, is for a very few specialised residential establishments. Therefore, work is underway to identify what might be effective hybrids. The current list for the types of setting in the UK is shown in Figure 1.1 and comprises:

- children's homes;
- boarding schools;
- hostels for refugee children;
- military training establishments (for young people under the age of 18);
- FE colleges;
- FE colleges for young people with special educational needs;
- special schools for cognition and learning difficulties;
- special schools for communication and interaction difficulties;
- special schools for sensory and/or physical difficulties;
- care homes for young people;
- hospital schools;
- children's hospices;
- psychiatric units;
- psychiatric units (forensic);
- young offender institutions;
- secure training centres;
- secure units;
- therapeutic communities;
- special schools for behavioural, emotional and social development difficulties.

In this inventory, which has been reviewed by staff in all sectors, the intention has been to distinguish the different types of setting by their major role. However, clear-cut distinctions are, in some cases, difficult to make, a point which is emphasised by the lengthy glossaries required in relevant government documents. Even with detailed definitions, some establishments still appear as hybrids while others seem to defy classification. For example, the children and young people in the special residential schools commonly exhibit more than one of the special educational needs (Cole, 1986). The issue is typified by a prospectus of one school in which it is stated that the school exists to help those special children and young people who experience autism and severe and complex

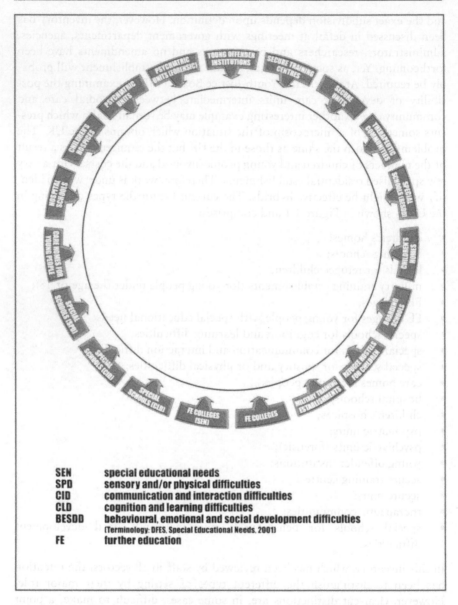

SEN   special educational needs
SPD   sensory and/or physical difficulties
CID   communication and interaction difficulties
CLD   cognition and learning difficulties
BESDD   behavioural, emotional and social development difficulties
         (Terminology: DFES, Special Educational Needs, 2001)
FE   further education

Figure 1.1   Residential and boarding education and care: types of setting

learning difficulties, and who exhibit associated challenging behaviour. A further result of attempting to simplify such a complexity of establishments is that some categories are groups with their own variation while others are well-defined types. For instance, the term 'children's homes' subsumes a variety of settings which house a range of children and young people with differing problems. In contrast, a secure training centre (STC), of which there are at present only three in the UK, is a precisely defined element in the secure estate.

A children's home is:

> an establishment (subject to certain exceptions) which provides care and accommodation wholly or mainly for children. Schools (both 'special' and 'mainstream') which accommodate children (e.g. as boarders) for more than 295 days a year.
>
> (DoH, 2002d)

The full definition is provided in the *Care Standards Act* (2000, Section 1). According to who runs them, whether or not they are for profit and with whom they need to be registered, the *Children Act* (1989) distinguishes between registered children's homes, voluntary homes and community homes (DoH, 1989b). With regard to the young people, some children's homes specialise but many may have, among others: children and young people whose families cannot cope, children and young people who have undergone multiply unsuccessful fosterings and young people on remand.

The term 'boarding schools' refers to mainstream schools, as distinct from special schools. Boarding schools are predominantly independent but there are thirty-four maintained boarding schools listed in the Stabis Guide (Stabis, 2003) plus a small number not listed. The number of schools which are totally boarding with full, as opposed to weekly, boarders is declining. While many children and young people are in boarding schools as a result of carefully considered decisions, it cannot be assumed that all have stable and united home backgrounds. A growing number have experienced disruption and have been exposed to potentially damaging and stressful experiences (Kahan, 1994). Children's homes and boarding schools were linked in Utting *et al.* (1997, Appendix C) which lists for 31 March 1996: 836 community homes run by local authorities, 64 voluntary children's homes, 202 registered (private) children's homes, 84 registered residential care homes and 40 independent schools registered as children's homes. Under the new definition in the *Care Standards Act* (2000), the number of such independent schools will have been greatly reduced. There are also international boarding schools throughout the world together with a number in the UK which specialise in taking foreign students (Findlay, 2000).

Hostels for refugee children and young people of all kinds are a recent development and support is available through the Refugee Council's Children's Panel. Since the issue of refugees is of growing concern, it seems likely that hostels will merit particular attention, and therefore they should be included as a separate type of setting in the inventory. The only obvious guideline occurs in children's homes Standard 36 (DoH, 2002d):

> Children in homes which are refuges approved under the *Children Act* (1989) are looked after in accordance with these National Minimum

Standards, with only those adaptations essential in the home concerned as a result of its status as a refuge.

In the UK, the minimum age for entry into the Armed Services is 16 for young men and 17 for young women. These young people therefore come within the age range of the *Children Act* (1989) but their care is not governed by it. For the Army, there are training establishments which cater specifically for young people within the 16 to 18 age range. In the other two Services, trainees of that age are normally mixed with those who are over 18 years old.

FE colleges provide training and education for those beyond the school-leaving age of 16. A reasonable number of FE colleges offer accommodation of various kinds ranging from purpose-built study bedrooms on the campus to approved lodgings. Particular oversight needs to be given to the 16 to 18 age group for which National Minimum Standards have been published (DoH, 2002a). One group of FE colleges provides for young people with special educational needs. Each such college must have the ability to provide a learning environment that matches the requirements of the students, however complex (NATSPEC, 2001 and 2002). In the glossary for the FE college standards, a specialist college is defined as follows:

> A college accommodating students with disabilities who are provided with personal nursing care, thus required to register as a Care Home with the National Care Standards Commission under the *Care Standards Act*, 2000.

They may be classified as between FE colleges and care homes but they are sufficiently distinctive to be listed separately.

Special schools are also something of a hybrid since they need to combine the care of children and young people normally associated with children's homes with the education provided by boarding schools. These schools may be supported by local authorities in which case they are known as maintained, by the voluntary sector when they are called non-maintained and by the private sector when they are independent. They offer boarding education for children and young people considered, within the meaning of the *Education Act* 1993, to have emotional and behavioural difficulties together with those who have learning difficulties or physical difficulties requiring specialised care and teaching (Kahan, 1994). The classification adopted in this inventory is that set out as areas of need by the DfES (2001a):

- communication and interaction;
- cognition and learning;
- behavioural, emotional and social development;
- sensory and/or physical.

Care homes for young people are those which provide accommodation and nursing or personal care for young people aged 16 and 17 who have: physical disabilities, sensory disabilities, learning disabilities, autistic spectrum disorders, mental health problems, alcohol or substance misuse problems, HIV/AIDS, dual and/or complex multiple disabilities including those who are deafblind (DoH, 2002c).

Hospital schools are special schools maintained by local education authorities (LEAs) within the premises of a hospital (DfES, 2001b). In general, arrangements are more flexible than those applying to special schools and hospital schools are not under a legal obligation to offer the National Curriculum. There are also hospital teaching services for chronically ill children and young people who are hospital in-patients (McCormack, 1979). A discussion on children and young people in hospital, including those in long-stay care, is provided in Kahan (1994).

Children's hospices provide palliative care for those children and young people whose illness may no longer be curable. The aim is to provide the best quality of life taking into account physical, emotional and spiritual care (Robinson and Jackson, 1999). Hospices also provide family support, respite care and bereavement services (Jackson and Eve, 2002).

Some children and young people develop severe emotional and behavioural disorders which require care and treatment beyond that which may be found in a school or sometimes even local health care. Some need special schools while others are placed in NHS or private mental health units or hospitals. Standards for the services are set out in Finch et al. (2000). These standards are separate from those set out for the care and treatment of children and young people. The hybrid establishment between this type of setting and custodial care is provided by the psychiatric unit (forensic).

The secure estate comprises three types of establishment. Young offender institutions (YOI) cater for young people between the ages of 15 and 18, offer by far the majority of the secure placements and are almost all run by the Prison Service. STCs take young people between the ages of 12 and 15, although on occasion younger and older young people are accommodated. They represent a new development and are owned and managed by independent companies. Local Authority Secure Units (LASUs) are social services provision (Harris and Timms, 1993), and approximately 30 per cent of the places are taken by young people not subject to any criminal order. The three types of setting are described in full in Rose (2002).

Therapeutic communities are establishments in which the residential and the educational environments are fully integrated to provide psycho-therapeutic treatment for exceptionally emotionally damaged young people. Legally, such communities may be classified as children's homes or, in certain cases, nursing homes or health care establishments. The Charterhouse Group (2001), which includes the main providers in this category, has produced a list of standards which apply in addition to those officially published for children's homes.

Therapeutic communities are considered sufficiently distinct from children's homes to be entered separately in the inventory.

All the types of setting listed may be considered residential although, in many of them, some of the children or young people may be only temporarily accommodated. The benefits of residential living and learning have long been recognised in a number of reports and publications (e.g. Davis, 1982, Scottish Office, 1992, Wagner, 1988) and, practically, by the provision of camps and short residential courses. The potential benefits of residential and boarding education and care are discussed in international settings (e.g. Gottesman, 1991), while, in the UK, residence is an important aspect of higher education (Brothers and Hatch, 1971). In the Children's Homes Regulations (2001), included in DoH, (2002d), the issue of permanence is specifically addressed among the excepted establishments:

> any establishment providing accommodation for children for less than twenty-eight days in any twelve month period in relation to any one child for the purposes of:
>
> (i)   a holiday; or
> (ii) recreational, sporting, cultural or educational activities.
>
> Such accommodation may be listed as adventure and activity centres.
> (Children's Placement Finder, 2004)

A further related category but one not included in the inventory for obvious reasons is mother-and-baby units. The children may be residential but they are not, of course, extra-familial.

Differences between the types of setting include the numbers of children and young people involved, the average size of establishment, the selection criteria and, in particular, whether the setting tends to be chosen or is a place for referral. Numbers in many of the types of setting are subject to rapid change or are, for other reasons, difficult to obtain. Broadly speaking, there are about 75,000 children and young people in mainstream boarding schools, approximately 20,000 in special residential schools and possibly as many again in FE colleges. In contrast, there are only a few hundred young people in secure training centres, secure units, therapeutic communities, hospices, psychiatric units and psychiatric units (forensic). For a stay of some three months, there are almost 3,000 children and young people in hospital schools, much the same number as there are in young offender institutions. There are about 7,000 young people in military training establishments, much the same number as in children's homes. The numbers in refugee hostels and care homes for young people are difficult to assess but probably amount to hundreds rather than thousands. The fact that in some types of setting the numbers change frequently is attributable to completion of whatever kind of treatment was undertaken but also, of course, the fact that when young people reach 18 years of age they pass outside the direct jurisdiction of the *Children Act* (1989) and are therefore not included in the statistics relevant for this book.

The different types of setting can be subdivided, according to the basic reason for residence, into four sectors: education, health, social and custodial (Figure 1.2). The first three sectors have long been associated together but it is

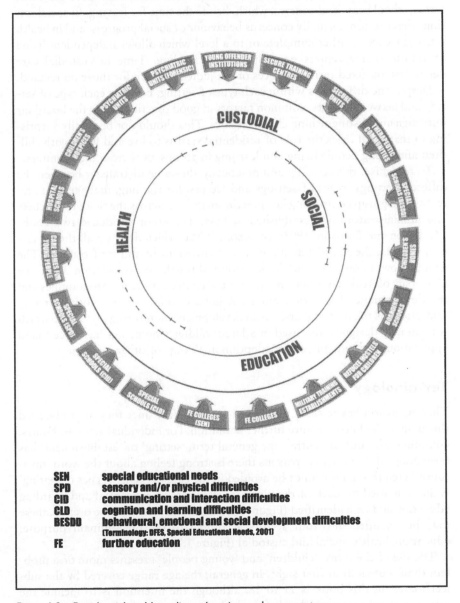

SEN	special educational needs
SPD	sensory and/or physical difficulties
CID	communication and interaction difficulties
CLD	cognition and learning difficulties
BESDD	behavioural, emotional and social development difficulties
	(Terminology: DFES, Special Educational Needs, 2001)
FE	further education

Figure 1.2   Residential and boarding education and care: sectors

only recently that the fourth sector has come under the *Children Act* (1989) and can be included. Apart from function, the sectors may be distinguished in a variety of ways, among the more obvious of which are the key characteristics of the children and young people and the criterion for leaving. In contrast to those in education, the children and young people in the other three sectors are likely to be relatively seriously disabled or damaged. In education, there are fixed terms, school years and courses, which dictate the time for leaving. In social settings the criterion normally concerns behaviour or social progress, and in health settings recovery, either complete or to a level which allows independent living or return to day centres or mainstream schooling. Time in custodial care depends upon fixed-term sentences or the judicial system for those on remand.

Despite the differences within each type of setting, between each type of setting and between sectors, common factors in good practice across the board far outweigh any distinguishing characteristics. This should not be totally surprising in that in all cases the role of residential staff is to live and work with children and young people living and learning in groups away from their families.

To recognise, theoretically and practically, the value of transfer between the different settings, types of settings and sectors, for training, management and research, a group comprising key practitioners from across the field, researchers and administrators was established in 1989. The group produced two books (Anderson and Davison, 1993; Anderson, 1994a) which drew on all the expertise to discuss the residential and boarding environment and staff training. The group, now known as the York Group through its association with the University of York, continues with research seminars, research programmes and the development of generic training. A good example of the work currently undertaken is the personal and social development monitoring procedure which was initially designed and used in a large children's home but has since found application, and in many cases, adoption in a range of other settings.

Terminology

This discussion has raised a number of terms which, since they are to be used throughout the book, require further definition. For individual schools, homes, communities, units or centres, the general term 'setting' or 'establishment' has been adopted. For obvious reasons there is strong feeling about the word 'institution' even though it cannot be avoided in the case of YOIs. 'Types of setting' is the term used for each of the nineteen categories of residential and boarding education and care identified (Figure 1.1). Although there is some overlap, these may be classified into four sectors according to the predominant purpose: education, health, social and custodial (Figure 1.2).

The use of the terms 'children' and 'young people' presents more of a problem than is obvious at first sight. In general, the age range covered by the subject matter in this book is 11 to 18, although the intention is to include the interests of preparatory schools for which the age range is commonly 7 to 13.

Exactly when children become young people is debatable, but it is generally taken to be at the age of 13 or 14. Ideally, the change might be linked to the onset of puberty or the start of adolescence, but these terms are also controversial. However, in general parlance, all those under the age of 18 are young people, including children. Children of 11 would hardly be offended to be designated young people but those of 17 would certainly not consider themselves children. The term 'children' is, of course, unavoidable in certain circumstances in that it is already part of the terminology, as in *Children Act* (1989), a children's home and child protection. In general, throughout the book the term 'young people' is preferred as a generalisation.

The other term commonly used in the book is considerably more contentious. What is the distinction between 'residential' and 'boarding' education? Generally, residential and boarding education and care is used since it covers both terms and the obvious functions. Care can be taken to subsume both social care and health care. One distinction is clear from the words themselves. Boarding implies 'boarding out' and, as a result, might be considered less permanent. The boarder's family residence is home whereas in residential education the setting is the residence. However, boarding may continue for seven years or more whereas most periods of residence are considerably shorter, some two months or even less. Boarding applies, of course, not only to mainstream schools but also to special boarding schools and both were subsumed under the title 'boarding schools' in the statistical appendage to *People Like Us* (Utting *et al.*, 1997). In that volume, boarding schools are listed as independent boarding schools, maintained boarding schools, independent special boarding schools approved by the Secretary of State, LEA special residential schools, non-maintained special residential schools and independent boarding schools also registered as children's homes. A distinguishing factor of boarding is that the length of residence normally relates directly to an external factor, education, and is according to standard school terms. There is also a closer partnership with families than in several of the other types of setting.

In contrast, residential education usually implies a continuous period from entry until leaving or release. Certainly, developments in mainstream boarding schools including weekly boarding and flexi-boarding emphasise the temporary nature of the stay in that type of setting. The period of residence is underlined by the *Care Standards Act* (2000) in which an establishment which accommodates one child for over 295 days in a year needs to register as a children's home.

The problem of definition concerning residential and boarding education and care is paralleled by that of the staff who live and work in the establishments. In the UK the wide variety of terms used includes: residential social worker, residential care staff, care staff, housemaster, housemistress, house parents, training staff and support staff. In continental Europe the social pedagogue is defined as the person who lives with the young people, teaches them and learns from them and with them. No such common term has arisen in the UK. Since there is great variation among the different types of setting not only as to the term used but also as to the job description, all staff who work in a caring role within the residence are referred to in this volume as 'residential staff'. They are the staff who have direct responsibility for the care of the young people living in the setting. They may not, and in most cases do not, live in themselves, and the term is used to distinguish them from those members of staff whose primary concern is health, education, administration or domestic and related duties.

An obvious question is: Why do the young people come into residence or boarding? There would appear to be four main reasons:

1   special provision is found in only a limited number of settings;
2   there is no accessible or fixed home;
3   to protect the public;
4   because residence is considered beneficial.

Using these as criteria, custodial care together with any setting which has young people on remand is clearly distinct and within the third category, although individual young people may still fit into any of the other three categories. Boarding schools are likely to include young people in all the remaining three categories. In health settings, residence may be due to the extreme or rare nature of the illness because of the general lack of specialised medical provision or, in a few cases, to protect the public. The social sector includes more of those young people who for whatever reason have no obvious home and grades towards the third category, protection of the public, since it includes young people on remand and some who have behavioural, emotional and social development difficulties.

As used in this volume, the term 'model' also merits some discussion. It is generally recognised that the word 'system' refers to a selected part of the real world, and systems theory as applied to organisations is particularly well analysed in Silverman (1970). A model is constructed to simplify this system with a view to enhancing understanding and facilitating prediction. The operation of the model can be tested by comparing the results it yields with those obtained in the real world.

The residential and boarding education and care system is extremely complex, and therefore it seems appropriate to construct and develop a model using the key variables selected logically, following a search of the relevant literature, from empirical observation and as a result of pilot studies. Given the data available, the most appropriate type is the intuitive model which can be subdivided in this case into morphological, cascading and process–response models. The morphological model comprises the structure through which energy, in the form of the cascading system, moves. The effect of the movement is to alter the morphology while the morphology itself governs the way the energy moves. Therefore, the two react together in what may be considered a process–response model. The operation can be governed by the introduction of a control model.

An analogy to illustrate this functioning can be taken from hydrology. A slope may be envisaged as a morphological model in which the major components such as soil depth, soil texture, moisture content and distance from the watershed are measured and related. When rainfall occurs, some remains on the surface, some infiltrates into the soil and flows through it, and some percolates into the rock below. This is the energy cascade. It may be seen that the movement of water on the surface or through the soil is strongly influenced by the slope factors while itself modifying both of them. For example, the rate of surface wash is governed by the slope gradient but erosion by water will eventually change the angle of the slope. A control might be represented by a wall at the base of the slope.

In terms of the residential and boarding education and care system, the morphological model would include the physical environment and the social structure including policies and procedures. The energy or cascading model is introduced into the system through the interaction of the staff, young people and visitors. In a process–response model, this human interaction is governed by the morphology but also moulds the structure to increase effectiveness of practice. A control would include the legal requirements for the operation of the system.

These four interrelated models provided the foundation upon which the model, the basis for this book, was originally constructed. However, it was considered that the process response idea might describe the relationship between the formal structure and the interactions of the staff and young people but did not sufficiently take into account the time elements such as the development of the young people and their transitions through the setting. As the development of the model is described in the following section, it will be seen that the morphological, cascading and process–response models refer to the environmental components and the control model to the framework components. The internal dynamics and interrelationships of these four sets of components allow analysis and interpretation of the entire system so that key elements may be identified, as appropriate, for practitioners, managers and researchers. Allied to this approach and of particular relevance to the developmental components but of application elsewhere, input/output models have been introduced.

At the simplest level, young people come into the establishment and leave it. If there is little indication as to what factors within the system result in their development, it is almost impossible to improve results. The system is then referred to as a 'black box', although this term may be modified if, through its basic characteristics, the model can be located on the family model-to-formal-model continuum (Robinson, 1994). As subsystems are identified and their effectiveness appraised, results can be improved and the black box is designated a 'grey box'. The aim is, of course, to have a 'white box' but light grey is perhaps a more realistic objective.

The model

Given the clear commonalities between the nineteen types of setting, the aim has been to produce a comprehensive generic model which could be used to develop ideas and practice and which would be capable of theoretical and practical application. It would describe basically what happens in all settings and summarise the key components. In this book, the components of the model and its application are described. Initial strands for the model were already in place in that the human and physical environments had been discussed and criteria for assessment trialled (Anderson and King, 1994). By implication, the external environment had been added in that there was particular concern in the work of the York Group for the issue of family relationships to be included. A number of profiles for the development of the young people were already recognised, as obviously were the controls produced by the *Children Act* (1989) and later legislation. There was general agreement that residential and boarding education and care focused upon the three main subjects of health, care and education. Residential living and residential establishments are the subject of continuity and change and therefore the time factor is clearly important. These variables were considered in different ways until a model emerged which not only summarised the key components and their relationships effectively but allowed the generation of new ideas.

The environmental components (Figure 1.3) were already clear in that the core of any setting is the human environment, the interaction between staff and young people. This is influenced in various ways by the built environment and other aspects of the surroundings which can together be designated the physical environment. As far as possible, the physical environment is gradually moulded to the requirements of the human environment but it none the less exercises some constraints which limit the activities which can take place. While the human and physical environment are clearly superimposed one upon the other for convenience, they are separated diagrammatically in the model.

However, the two together are not an isolated system in that, most important, there are family relationships and, as far as possible, a partnership between the establishment and those with parental responsibility in the upbringing of the young people. In addition, external expertise ranging from counsellors and doctors to therapists or independent visitors is required. Physically, the environment is also not isolated in that there are likely to be influences from and ideally a beneficial relationship with the local community. On a regional and national scale, there will also be inputs including inspections and all the legal requirements. Since they are external to the living and learning environment, all these influences have been grouped as the external environment.

The external environment may impinge upon the setting to a greater or lesser degree and this is indicated by the position of the chevron (Figure 1.3). For example, in boarding schools the chevron may effectively bisect the human and physical environment, indicating that there is a very close relationship between

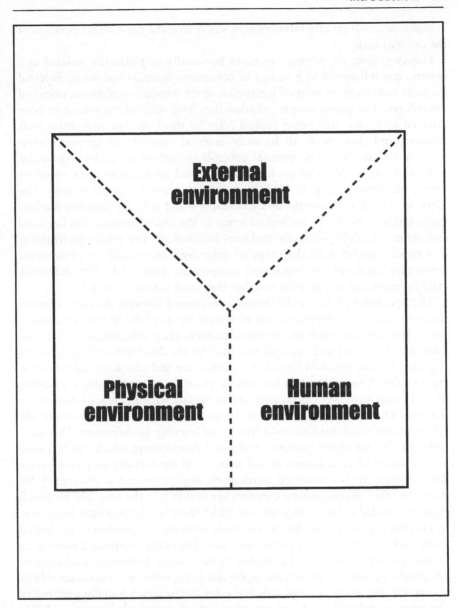

Figure 1.3   **Environmental components**

the external environment and the establishment. Indeed, the public may use facilities and share in events to such an extent that the only private areas are the dormitories and bedrooms. In a secure setting, parental contact may be far more intermittent and may indeed impose some form of risk for the young people. In that case, the chevron would be very shallow. The three environmental components, in their interrelationships, summarise the day-to-day operation of the establishment.

However, since the setting can never be socially or physically isolated as a system, it is influenced by a variety of constraints upon its operation. External controls stem from an array of legislation which imposes regulations, rules and procedures. The young people, whether they have selected the setting or been referred to it, are still being looked after by third parties away from their families, and there needs to be some external oversight to guarantee their security and welfare. The internal controls are subsumed under philosophy, aims and ethos. The philosophy sets the broad path, possibly in visionary terms, which the setting should follow, and is expressed in terms of aims. The aims set out clear directions and destinations and it is the progress towards these which gives rise to the feel or ethos of the establishment. The key legal constraints are child protection and non-discrimination or equal opportunities and these, together with the range of other legal issues and the philosophy/ aims/ethos, constitute the framework components (Figure 1.4). They frame the establishment and its operations in that they exert ultimate control.

The operation of the establishment is expressed through the interaction of the environmental components but within the limits of the framework components. However, there will be constant changes as the young people develop, and these are monitored and assessed according to the developmental components (Figure 1.5). The common threads are health, care and education, all defined in the broadest terms. Health is not merely about medicine but about a healthy lifestyle while care includes security and increasing self-sufficiency. Education is not only what happens in school or classroom but includes the lessons of life which accrue from residence in a living and learning environment. This environment also influences personal and social development which can be evaluated in terms of such factors as self-esteem and the forming of relationships. This component is considered particularly important and is distinguishable from the other developmental components in that it is the only one for which there are no dedicated settings and for which there is relatively little in the way of external expertise available. It is in many ways the end product of residential living. What kind of young person emerges? The other component thought to be particularly important is behaviour. In this context behaviour is taken to lie on a bad-to-good continuum, the aggregate being taken to be unacceptable or acceptable. For many settings, this is the key factor which initially gave rise to the entry or referral of the young person. Such specific behaviour is distinguished from behaviour which indicates what people do in any situation and is used to assess progress.

Time (Figure 1.6) brings change, planned or inadvertent, and may be subdivided in any way required. It is distinguished in the model by using a short time frame, daily living, and, the longest for the young person, transitions from pre-entry to post-leaving. The analogy of the model is with a filing system, and the environmental and framework components are on each card from the first,

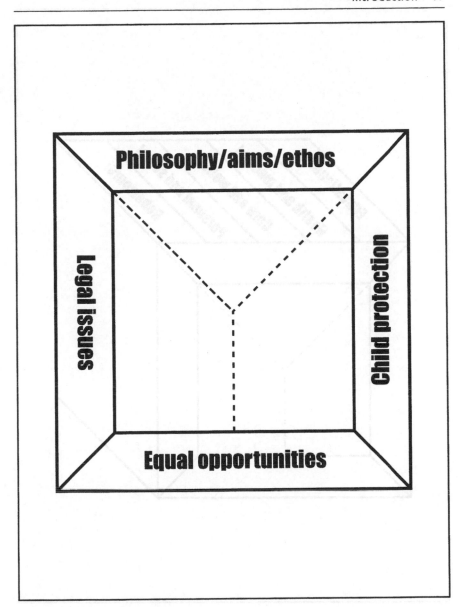

Figure 1.4 Framework components

which represents the present back through the system to the point of entry. The developmental components are traced along the filing system from the back card to the front, current, card. Time is taken as a twenty-four-hour period, the thickness of the card, and transitions extend from before the entry card through to the future.

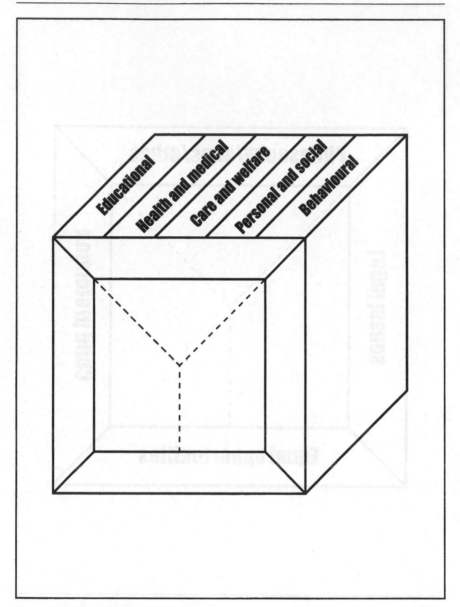

Figure 1.5   Developmental components

The four components together comprise the model which provides a summary of residential and boarding life and has application for training, management and research (Figure 1.7). For whatever reason the book is used, the core
concern remains the needs of young people in the living and learning environment. Each set of components provides a different viewpoint upon this concern.

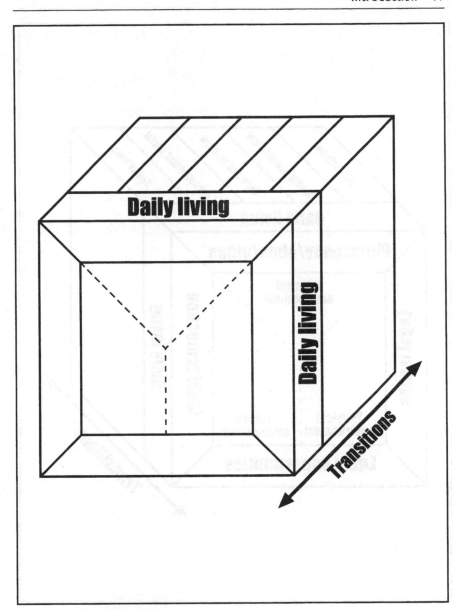

Figure 1.6   Time components

The environmental components set out the major factors which comprise the living and learning environment while the framework components consider the guidelines which influence its operation. The developmental components examine the progress of the young people towards their needs, and the time components cover the basic unit of time and the fundamental changes which occur in

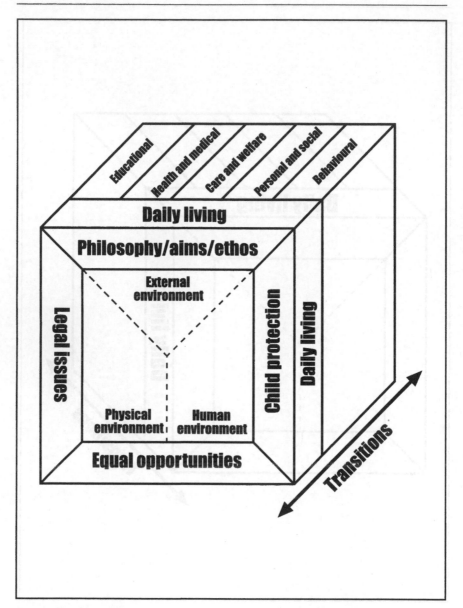

Figure 1.7   The model

the young people throughout their association with the setting. At the same time, the intention is that each set of components should be discussed in full as a complete entity. In attempting to provide a common focus but also complete coverage, there is necessarily some overlap and repetition. For example, residential or boarding education is important in considering both the human environment and the use of staff time. Parental responsibility needs to be examined as the key part of the external environment but also as a legal issue. Care for the young people is a developmental component and a legal requirement.

In social work in general there is increasing evidence upon the provision of research-based evidence to inform evidence-based practice (e.g. Ward, 1995). In residential and boarding education and care research is limited, and it is one hope behind this book that more will be stimulated. As far as possible, guidance on practice has been supported by research findings but, inevitably, much of the evidence has to be drawn from recognised good practice and guidelines from analogous situations.

Chapter 2

Environmental components

The purpose of residential and boarding education and care is to fulfil, as far as possible in an ex-familial situation, the needs of a particular group of young people. To achieve this purpose, each setting has an environment which is specialised in terms of education, health, social care, custodial care, or any combination of these to address the specific needs. The key elements of the environment are the young people and those who fulfil the main nurturing role, the residential staff. The environment is also characterised by the management and support staff, the factors of specialisation including grounds, buildings, facilities, equipment and staff and visitors, especially the families of the young people. Together, these constitute the living and learning environment peculiar to a particular setting. Since behaviour, taken in a general sense, is a function of personality and environment, the characteristics of the complete setting are obviously vital for the development of the young people. The environmental components therefore encapsulate the core of residential and boarding education and care.

For experienced practitioners, the overall environment is apparent in the ambience or feel of the establishment. While this is clearly subjective, depending upon the past experience and preferences of the observer, there are many indicators which build up, subconsciously, a total picture. Among these may be the way residential staff treat the young people, the relationship between the young people and the domestic staff, the state of the decorations and furnishings, the ambient conditions in the public rooms and the level of attention given to the gardens and grounds. The mood can change from day to day but this does not affect the overall ethos. An analogy might be with weather and climate in that the former represents short, sharp, transient changes whereas the latter indicates underlying trends. It is clear that the ethos, as the product of philosophy and aims, should be congruent with equal opportunities, child protection and other key legal issues.

If the young people coming into residence are to be matched with an appropriate setting, it is important that there is a detailed understanding of the environment. Although the establishments within any type of setting are likely to have many variables in common, each is unique. The Dartington Social

Research Unit has attempted to capture this characteristic for children's homes in terms of structure and culture and the effect on outcome (Brown *et al.*, 1998; Bullock *et al.*, 1999). The basic characteristics of homes are identified in Sinclair and Gibbs (1996). Anderson and King (1994) distinguish between the physical and the social environment while Kahan (1994) includes in a chapter on the physical environment, a section entitled 'The environment as a whole: the feel of the place'. From the research perspective, it is clearly difficult to develop measures which are both reliable and valid but even an inventory of key environmental factors would represent a significant improvement in the possibilities for the appropriate placement of the young people.

For the practitioner wishing to operate effectively in the environment, it is vital to develop an understanding of the important elements. What is the policy governing the relationships between the young people? How are the values of the establishment demonstrated in the environment? (DoH, 1989a). What are the pastoral roles of the senior members of staff? Where are the key service controls such as those for water and electricity located? Is access to parts of the establishment limited? How are the surroundings used? Under what conditions are the young people allowed beyond the boundaries?

The identification of key elements may be approached in a variety of ways. Using a topic-based approach, a subject such as relationships might be selected. It clearly covers relationships between staff and other staff, staff and young people, staff and visitors, staff and external experts, and families and young people. Relationships need to be initiated, sustained and, at times, ended. Such a systematic approach could also be used to include subjects such as: group dynamics, intervention, conflict resolution, staff training, the monitoring of visits, the use of experts, problems with the buildings or services and emergency procedures. Another approach could be termed 'spatial'. In this the internal aspects of the setting, including the young people, staff and buildings, could be distinguished from the grounds and local surroundings and the external environment.

More effectively, if the two procedures are combined, a distinction of applied value may be made between the three basic environments:

1   human or social;
2   physical, particularly built;
3   external (Figure 2.1).

Any division of the total environment is artificial and there are obvious overlaps between the three aspects identified. Indeed, for practical purposes the human and physical environments are separated in the model but, in life, one is superimposed upon the other. However, it does seem logical to distinguish the human activity from the physical setting in which it takes place. It is also reasonable to limit the human environment to those who normally live and work within the establishment and to designate all influences predominantly from outside as the external environment. Within each of the three environments, a systematic

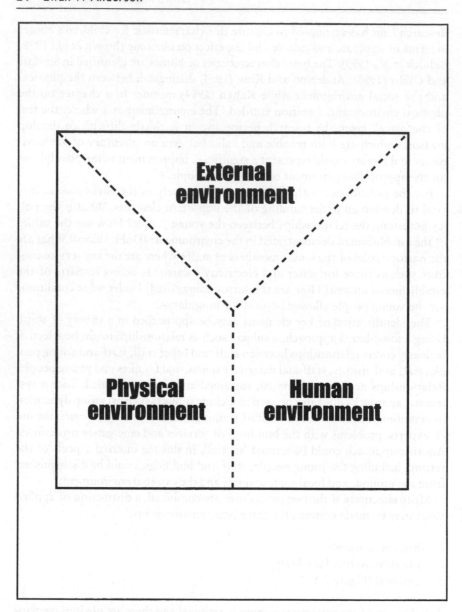

Figure 2.1   Environmental components

approach may then be adopted. The distinction can be justified in that, for example, relationships within the human environment between staff and young people who are effectively living together and those between members of the resident community and those who live and work mostly away from it are likely to be different.

For the inexperienced practitioner, the human environment is the most important, together with those aspects of the physical environment which influence active participation in emergencies and important procedures. Staff development entails a deepening knowledge of the human environment, an increasingly detailed appreciation of the physical environment and its effects, and a developing collaboration with the external environment.

It is an informative exercise to consider the degree of fit between the three environments. In general terms, the human environment fits closely to the physical environment. For all the human activities of the establishment, the range of rooms, buildings and grounds need to be used. However, wear and tear, pressures and tensions can all indicate that the human environment is over-fitting and more space is required. Such a situation arises, for example, where specialist residential provision is needed. Some health facilities and many units within the custodial care sector are either overcrowded or the facilities cannot hope to meet demand. In some cases there will be an under-fit, a common occurrence when an establishment is declining. The situation may vary over time. For example, a small children's home can change rapidly from under-fit to over-fit. These considerations raise the important issue of the margin on which the establishment operates. In a climate in which cost-effectiveness is rated very highly, an empty bed represents a significant loss of revenue. Boarding schools have declined somewhat in numbers over the past twenty years and one solution has been to convert the specialised boarding units for other school purposes and to enhance the number of day pupils. For mainstream and special schools in more isolated areas, the introduction or expansion of the day population may not be a realistic possibility.

More obvious mismatches occur between the human environment and the external environment (Figure 2.2). Assuming that privacy for the young people is a key issue and visitors, even professionals, are limited in their access, no element of the external environment will completely coincide with the human environment. In the case of health care settings, the need for specialist medical provision may mean that there is a close match between the two environments. In custodial care, the need for security is likely to restrict the incursion of the external environment. An interesting example is that of family relationships and visits. In some boarding schools parents may have access to virtually the complete human environment since family influence is considered beneficial. In custodial care settings in which, in some cases, the effects of the family may be thought potentially harmful, the access will be extremely limited. If it is assumed that the more open the establishment, the less the chance of abuse or other such problems, then the question of the overlap of the external with the human and therefore the physical environments is of great relevance.

The entire issue of the interrelationships between the three environments is, of course, central to any mechanism for matching and routes into residential and boarding education and care. The matching process is essentially generated in the external environment and is, in many settings, controlled

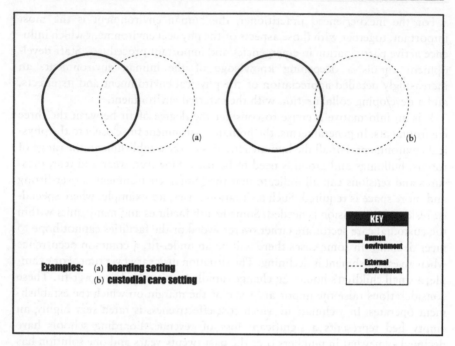

Figure 2.2   Human and external environments

from that environment (Dartington Social Research Unit, 2001). For example, in the secure estate, the arrival of the young people is conditioned primarily by the need for residential accommodation rather than anything specific about the actual setting and it may be pure fortune whether a young person comes into an LASU, an STC or a YOI (Rose, 2002). Since these units are likely to be run respectively by the Local Authority, a private company and the Prison Service and, given the differences between them in scale and staffing, the environments are quite distinctive. In special schools and boarding schools, while the decision is made externally by those with parental responsibility, open days are now a common feature and discussion is encouraged with the school staff on the suitability of the environment. In FE colleges and military establishments the choice is usually that of the young person. Therapeutic communities have, through experience, developed an inventory of criteria for the selection of the young people. It is only for young adults in care homes that the need for preliminary visits is a standard requirement. However, throughout residential and boarding education and care the budget for each establishment depends upon a certain level of occupancy, and in most settings criteria for entry are not absolutely rigid. Public–private initiatives reinforce the business-based approach.

Apart from the degree of superimposition of the three environments, there is clearly interaction between them. The physical environment can constrain the activities within the human environment but may also suggest additional pro-grammes. For example, there may be no swimming pool but there may be a nearby lake which can be used for fishing and sailing. The most obviously and purposely constrained physical environment is that of a custodial care setting where freedom of movement is limited in the interests of security. However, it is possible to organise room use and programmes so that every view is not of a high wall surmounted by razor wire. Thus, the physical environment or its effects may be modified to fit the human environment and vice versa. The two environments present an example of a process–response system in that each influences the other, and activities are affected by the environment but may also modify it.

The physical environment interacts with the external environment in that it presents a boundary and some level of check upon entry. In the case of board-ing schools, the constraint may only be upon those who do not live there enter-ing the dormitories and living accommodation. However, given the problems of intruders and the requirements of child protection, most establishments for young people have developed a security system involving one, or at most a few, entry points and the identification of visitors by badges. However, boundaries vary in porosity both for entry and exit. There are obviously other interactions through the provision of services and maintenance of the physical environment. The human environment reacts with the external environment through the net-work of visitors ranging from families or those with parental responsibility to counsellors, social workers, medical staff and other specialist professionals. Furthermore, young people in all but the custodial care sector are likely to make regular use of the locality of the establishment. Many of the staff will live near the setting and there may well be support for activities both inside and outside the establishment.

Since the total environment is produced by the interaction of the three envi-ronmental components, this interplay will affect all aspects of the development of the young people as illustrated by the developmental components (Chapter 4). Education may be external to the setting or in the internal environment, where it is bound to be affected by the physical environment. It is commonly external in children's homes, care homes for young people and hostels for refugee children. Health and medical provision may be focused in the establish-ment but will normally require significant external inputs. Care and welfare is located in all settings but, in some cases, needs to draw heavily on the external environment. In boarding schools, there will normally be relatively little input from social workers but in most of the other settings their support will be sig-nificant. Behaviour management is largely an internal concern but there may be key external inputs, particularly in settings concerned primarily with some approach to behaviour modification. Personal and social development is the only developmental component which is virtually exclusively internal. However, even in this case there is likely to be some enhancement from outside, for example, from visitors and through excursions.

The division of the environment into three components facilitates analysis and understanding. It also allows a number of interesting assessments to be made such as the degree of openness of the establishment. The subdivision also helps elucidate considerations for training, management and research. The reduction of complexity entailed in discussing each component separately allows a clearer understanding of the interactions at each level and between the three environments. Although the subdivision is essentially artificial, it can be justified for the purposes of matching young people and the environment and of making effective comparisons between different settings.

Human environment

The human environment is taken to comprise two elements:

1   the young people in residence; and
2   the staff who work regularly within the establishment.

There are clearly many professionals who work within the setting for limited periods but they, together with all visitors including those from the family are, for the purposes of analysis, considered to be part of the external environment. For example, a doctor may visit once or twice a week and a counsellor may attend on a regular basis but they are in essence external. In a children's hospital, of course, a doctor working with the young people in residence on a daily basis would be part of the human environment. The human environment is produced by the interaction of those who live and work within the physical environment of the establishment on a regular basis. It is they who provide the self-sufficient aspect of the setting.

For the young people, the distinction is fundamentally according to whether they sleep in the establishment. However, some boarding schools have extended day pupils who take most meals in school and may stay until late evening. Although they do not have the commitment of living in, if they are attached to boarding houses or residential units, they, like those staff who work but do not live in the establishment, must be included as part of the human environment. Boarding however provides some interesting issues with regard to definition, as, for example, with those who board occasionally with a flexi-boarding scheme under which they can sign in for an overnight stay. Furthermore, it must be realised that in certain settings many young people are short-stay. A major difficulty in assessing the number of young people in hospital schools is that the population changes so frequently. Similarly, in many children's homes there are few long-term residents. The current Detention and Training Order (DTO) specifies only two months of custodial care.

Some staff members may also live within the establishment and indeed, in boarding, this is the norm. In special schools, house staff were normally residential but, as a result of costs and problems of recruitment, members on duty now commonly 'sleep in', on a rota basis, rather than live in. In many ways this is an unfortunate development in that having families living in the establishment must be beneficial for the young people. However, there is a view that the effects of residence on families and, particularly the children of staff, may be potentially harmful. Certainly, in situations where there are, for whatever reason, serious behavioural problems among the young people, children of staff may not be in actual danger but their development may be affected. The fact remains that if one of the benefits of residence is the presence of staff as models, then the decline of family living within settings must be considered a retrograde step.

In all the settings, the majority of staff are likely to live externally. They may enter the human environment as teachers, administrative staff or domestic staff for the normal working day or they may be on a shift system. In dealing with particularly damaged young people, some establishments have night patrols and the night staff can be only marginally part of the human environment interaction although they are often there at critical times (Farmer and Pollock, 1998). All core staff of whatever kind contribute in some way to the human environment and therefore have potential to support the development of the young people.

The fundamental ambience of the establishment in which the two groups interact to produce the human environment should relate to the values and aims of the setting (see Chapter 3), possibly modified by the physical environment. There are many sources for the aims and values. They may have been developed over many years or they may, as in several celebrated cases, result from the beliefs of one director or principal. The work of A. S. Neill at Summerhill (Walmsley, 1969) immediately springs to mind. However they originated, the aims and values are likely to undergo change or at least amendment as society itself changes. There may well remain underlying eternal verities but the way they are expressed will alter over time. For example, a major purpose must be to prepare the young people for independent living in current society. How much should this requirement be allowed to affect the aims? Clearly the establishment must have standards, but how will the future life of the young people be affected if these standards clash with those of society? For many of the young people leaving several of the settings, particularly those in the custodial care sector, survival in life is difficult enough without the handicap of having been prepared for living under conditions which no longer exist. Therefore, while the need to inculcate such aims as honesty, selflessness and virtue might be considered unchanging, they must be set in the context of the modern world. These issues must be seen in the context of a world in which many parents effectively relinquish responsibility for moral and spiritual training and in which religious studies in schools, formerly employed as a source of values and standards, have been diluted. Whether these changes can be adequately compensated by lessons in citizenship must be at best conjectural.

A summary diagram of the human environment is set out in Figure 2.3. To simplify matters, all inputs from the external environment have been omitted.

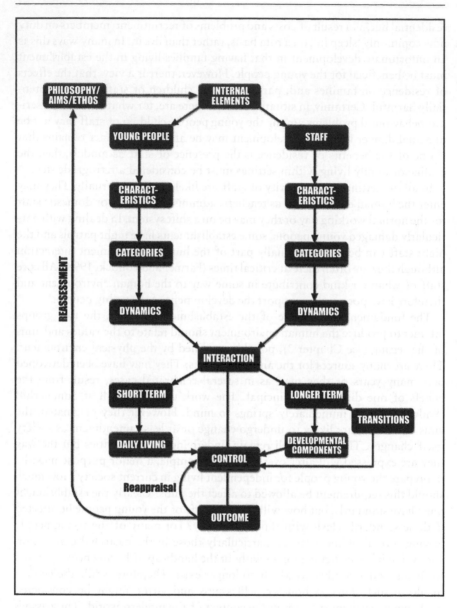

Figure 2.3   Human environment

The internal elements comprise the young people and the staff, each with distinguishing categories and characteristics. Both groups have their own internal dynamics and the interaction of the two provides the core of the human environment. The effects of this interaction are seen, in the short term, in all the aspects of daily living and, in the longer term, through the developmental components and the transitions through which each young person can pass. Controls are exercised over this interaction and the result may be described as the outcome for the establishment, the staff and the young people. Since many of the controls involve legislation, the outcome needs to be reappraised against them. The outcome is also reassessed in the light of the philosophy, aims and ethos of the establishment so that any necessary adjustments may be made. For example, if the outcome with regard to the young people appears to be in some way ineffective, this may be as a result of the young people, their categories and characteristics or their relationships. It may be as a result of the staff but in both cases the selection of individuals may be governed from outside or for some other reason difficult to change. In any case, it is more likely that the remedy will be found in the interaction between the staff and young people ranging from intervention through the variety of programmes to pastoral care. It is also possible that the problem may relate to the system of control and the way it is exercised, although this should have become apparent through the reappraisal procedure. In the following sections, each element of the model is examined and discussed.

Young people: characteristics

A suitable inventory of the characteristics of young people living away from home in groups is: needs; age; capabilities; mix; numbers; behaviour; and skill levels. Of particular relevance is the degree of variation within each of these characteristics. All young people have basic needs but some have needs beyond these which are specific and which set them apart from their peers. These needs are likely to be concerned in some way with care, health, behaviour or education. The result for the human environment may be that staff are required to spend a disproportionate amount of time with certain individuals. This is a major issue which confronts the DfES in its dialogue with boarding schools about the possible placement of more young people with special educational needs. What types of need can be accommodated and how many young people can be introduced per unit before the character of the group is itself distorted? It depends very much upon the size of the group and the types of need currently being served. Sensory and/or physical difficulties may impose particular requirements upon the physical environment but, of all the needs, are probably most likely to elicit support from other members of the group.

Since the focus of community life is upon interaction and communication, those young people who have particular difficulties are in danger of remaining as isolates. Consequently, a great deal of staff time may be required for social engineering to ensure inclusion. Cognition and learning difficulties may affect the functioning of a group but are likely to be of most significance in the classroom. Depending upon the specifics of the case, young people with behavioural, emotional and social development difficulties are likely to be the most demanding of staff time and the most difficult to fit into groups. Depending on the size of group, a rule of thumb would be that only one such young person could be effectively assimilated.

Differences in age are to be expected, whether in a family group model of residence or in a formal model of boarding. However, from the staff viewpoint, marked differences in age produce potential problems in direct relation to the size of the group. In a small group, it is clearly easier to plan all aspects of life from education to therapy and leisure activities the closer the young people are in age. Whether or not differences in age actually increase the chances of abuse and bullying, the general perception is that they do. Under normal circumstances, an increase in all-round capabilities would be expected with advancing years. As the young people move from dependence to independence, their ability to look after themselves in all facets of life tends to grow. Marked variations in capability as in age or needs, all of which may be interrelated, can be potentially difficult for staff. The sum of such variables is the mix which expresses the variation in basic requirements.

The issue of numbers raises some interesting questions. What is the ideal size of unit or sub-unit? Is there a magic number which allows everyone to receive attention but no one to feel over-exposed? What are the appropriate staffing ratios? What limit does size place upon activities? In the research there is no generally accepted size of unit which has been shown to be the most beneficial. There is an interesting discussion on size in relation to school classes in Blatchford (2003). The only numbers which appear in the literature with any regularity are seven and twelve (e.g. Douglas, 1977). The approved staff to student ratio for external visits in mainstream schools is one to fifteen. Particularly small numbers for a residential group can lead to highly intense and possibly damaging relationships. Large numbers can result in neglect and failure to spot harmful developments. In the extreme, small numbers correspond with the family model and large numbers with the formal model, seen in military groupings or boarding schools before the modern period. Numbers are clearly of great importance but the actual significance depends upon the characteristics of the young people, the number of staff available and the intended activities. Berridge (1985) includes an interesting discussion in which he relates environmental factors to size in children's homes.

Smaller units nearer the family model end of the scale have many advantages in that all the functions have a well-defined focus and the staff and young people are likely to know each other well. Given the advantages of a relatively small size, larger settings commonly subdivide the population of young people into smaller groups often according to purpose. There may be further subdivision so that the establishment is effectively multi-sized (Figure 2.4).

Behaviour is closely related to needs and, within the human environment, the first consideration is whether the behaviour of an individual is, by normal standards, good or bad. The main point is how much staff attention or control is required. For example, it may be possible to manage either particularly deviant behaviour by one young person or a degree of poor behaviour by the whole

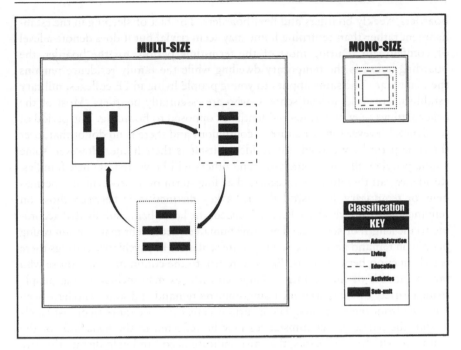

Figure 2.4   Size of unit

group but not both together. Skill levels are clearly linked to capabilities and are relevant to the activity being undertaken. For many activities, the skill levels of the young people will be known in advance and it will be possible to fashion groups, with regard to size and individual young people, according to staff competence.

These characteristics provide guidelines which describe any group of young people in the human environment. The more that is known about the young people, the more elaborate the classification can become. For example, the term 'mix' would take into account the full array of personal variables considered in any anti-discrimination policy (Millam, 1996), discussed in Chapter 3. Most importantly, these would include culture, gender, sexuality, ethnicity, language, disability and religion. Although related elements are covered in the inventory, the personality of each young person will be important in group engineering and activity. Some are more optimistic than others, and some will be more committed to the particular task. Some of these variables will be known in advance and others will emerge only during the course of residential living.

Young people: categories

There will also be variations among the young people in what, from the residential viewpoint, may be considered categories. In boarding, there may be full boarders, weekly boarders and flexi-boarders. The fact of sleeping in the establishment rather than returning home may seem trivial but it does denote a level of commitment. During most of the term-time period, for the boarder, the boarding house is the temporary dwelling while the family residence remains the real home. The same applies to young people living in FE colleges, military establishments and special schools, who are essentially boarders. Most of the other settings may be termed residential as opposed to boarding. The period of residence, however long or short, is continuous and there is no doubt that, over the time period concerned, the residence itself is their home. However, some young people will have home visits and others will be visited by their families. Residence can therefore be categorised as long-term or short-term and permanent or temporary. In custodial care, a key distinction is between those on remand and those who have been sentenced, the latter being subdivided according to the length of sentence. The same human environment may contain young people on remand and those serving a life sentence. In psychiatric settings there is a distinction between those likely to return to the community and those who face a lifetime of incarceration. Children's homes may include young people from a variety of categories including some on remand and some who have been removed from their parents. These various categories are more than just labels in that the particular circumstances may be reflected in the behaviour of the young people. In some cases, they also indicate needs and help dictate the care regime. As with the mix of characteristics, a generally homogeneous group is likely to lessen staff problems.

Young people: dynamics

The interactions within the group of young people, as opposed to those between the young people and the staff, are greatly influenced by the mix of characteristics (Blatchford, 1998). Each young person is linked to the group by communications and the development of relationships (Callow, 1993). This link between personal and social development is discussed in Chapter 4. Communications between the young people may be verbal or non-verbal and will be predominantly informal (Atherton, 1989). Some are better communicators in a general sense than others. Some will communicate more easily with their peers than with staff, a point which will become apparent only through careful observation and monitoring. Support needs to be provided to those who have difficulty in relating to others, if they are to gain the full benefits of residential education (Brown and Christie, 1981).

It is through relationships that social development occurs (Callow, 1993). The range of potential relationships obviously increases with the size of the group and the length of time in residence. If the period of stay is shorter than the integration period into the establishment, there are unlikely to be any relationships other than the most temporary and superficial. In a small family group of four or six young people, the characteristics may be so relatively disparate that there is little that each has in common with the others and any relationships are likely to be very loose. In situations where there can be a shared interest in the longer term, relationships may last for life. Young people who are residential in FE colleges undoubtedly have the greatest freedom socially. In a boarding school there may be shared activities, membership of the same house, form or team, or links may be developed as a result of common external circumstances. Military training may produce friendships which last throughout a military career. Except under special circumstances, friendships formed in children's homes, health settings and custodial care are less likely to survive the period of residence.

Relationships may also be negative. Among other factors, status differentials may result in abuse or bullying and staff need to be aware of the potential for unhealthy relationships. Since relationships clearly result from attraction, at some level, between individuals, the concern must be with the nature of that attraction and, for some types of attraction, how it is expressed. Among the more difficult to address are sexual relationships which are likely to seem extremely important to the participants and which, depending upon age, might be condoned elsewhere.

There is a general perception that, despite the potential benefits, living away from home in groups, whether as a result of choice or referral, represents a measure of deprivation. This may be reduced according to the mode of residence and in particular the strength of partnership between the establishment and the family. However, assuming some deprivation resulting from extra-familial living, residence and boarding can provide, by way of some compensation, the opportunity for strong bonding.

Since relationships are so important in the human environment (Stanley and Reed, 1999), it can be interesting and helpful to produce sociograms for each of the young people, or certainly those judged to be at risk, indicating their various links among their peers. Indeed, knowledge of peer group relationships provides a good indicator of the staff's understanding of the young people (Gahagan, 1975). Sociograms are particularly useful as a supervision or management tool in considering developmental problems.

The way the young people relate to each other, to the various groups and to the overall group is apparent not only in leisure pursuits and private time but also in the activities of the human environment. These include all the aspects of daily living together with programmes relating directly to development and formal or guided leisure pursuits. This interaction among the young people constitutes a significant part of residential education. There will be potential for cooperation but also conflict and conflict resolution. Peer group learning may occur in connection with formal education or learning for life. Academic problems may be best explained by a member of the peer group who has experienced the difficulties. Indeed, the basis of living together in a harmonious and reasonable fashion is probably best learned from peers. For this reason, the peer group has become a focus of study throughout residential and boarding education and care. Whether in children's homes, special schools or custodial care the peer group is highly significant for learning and preparation for later life. Post-residential success is likely to depend, in no small measure, upon the peer group, and therefore some reasonable level of integration with the peer group within residence is important (Cowie and Wallace, 2000).

Within any peer group which is established for more than a very short time, a pecking order emerges. For various reasons, some young people attain a higher status than others. Status may be acquired as a result of a large number of factors ranging from aspects of background to physical or mental variables. In animal groups, the physical appears to dominate and settlement of disputes is through conflict. For staff working with groups of young people, it is very important to know the source of status, since it may not accord with the values of the establishment and efforts may be required to change it. For example, in custodial care status may vary directly in relation to the seriousness of the offence. Clearly this flies in the face of practice which is to confront offending behaviour and for the offender to express remorse. In boarding schools, the factor giving status was traditionally sporting ability but this has been extended to include aspects of academic work, music, drama and art. However, personal characteristics may also play a key role. A good example is a sense of humour. Those who appear to have little such cultural currency, a term used to encapsulate status characteristics (Callow, 1994), may well be the target for bullying, not necessarily through violence but perhaps through neglect. They can also be isolates and it may require strong efforts by staff to develop strategies to help them integrate into groups.

Between the core members of a group and the isolates there may be some young people who may be characterised as 'knife-edgers' (Callow, 1994). Whether it is in the group or with staff, they do just enough to survive and maintain their own position. They pose particular problems for staff since their public behaviour is likely to be quite different from that which can occur in private. As a result, their performance and progress may be better judged by a cleaner than by a member of the residential staff.

Staff: characteristics

To work with each other and with the young people, staff characteristics must also be factored into the programme. The most basic is the number of staff usually expressed as the staffing ratio, a figure set out in legal documents for many of the settings. However, given the range of variables among the young people, some flexibility is required and recent research by the Residential Forum (2002) has resulted in a procedure for calculation which is accepted by the DoH. So far, this has been developed for younger adults in care homes but there would appear to be no reason why the principle should not be applied throughout residential and boarding education and care. This would provide recognition for the fact that some establishments require more staff time than others and that, even within one establishment, there may be marked variation among the units.

Calculation of the current staffing ratio depends very much upon which staff are included. If all staff are counted, the ratio in an STC is likely to be about three staff per young person. Ratios may be even higher in some psychiatric settings. However, in comparing ratios between the different sectors, it is not always clear that like is being compared with like. For example, in hospital schools, a high proportion of the staff may be concerned with the young people for only a very limited time span per day. In a boarding school, ratios appear very low, possibly one staff member for thirty or more young people. However, this calculation may include only the house staff who are officially delegated to boarding duties. Apart from the domestic staff and the matron, account should be taken of staff who work in the school but not specifically in the boarding house (Brandon *et al.*, 1998).

Other important characteristics include professional skills, training level and specialisms. There are also factors resulting from personality including motivation, self-perceptions and belief. The member of staff is not only a facilitator and guarantor of security but, most important, a model. Indeed, in residential or boarding education, or whatever the living and learning is styled, the fact that the staff act as models is thought to be crucial. Therefore, staff characteristics are vital whatever the type of establishment. According to their age, staff also bring a variety of life experiences to the human environment. Therefore, it is reasonable to think that whereas homogeneity among the young people is an advantage, among staff heterogeneity can be clearly beneficial. Certainly, the personal characteristics of the staff must be considered seriously when their deployment among the young people is planned.

Staff: categories

The most obvious categorisation of staff is according to function. Depending upon the type of establishment, staff may be classed as: residential, care, teaching, health, administrative, domestic, ancillary, grounds or external. Members of the different staff units will not necessarily all come into contact with the young people. All young people will need to interact with residential staff although in boarding schools such staff may also be teachers. Indeed, in boarding schools the young people are likely to encounter all the different categories listed. In health settings the young people may not meet administrative, domestic or grounds staff. In children's homes, the teaching staff are normally not attached to the home. In custodial care, it may be only the care and teaching staff together with some external professionals who are commonly encountered. Every member of staff who can possibly come into unsupervised contact with the young people not only requires clearance from the Criminal Records Bureau (CRB) but also needs to be aware of the aims and values of the establishment. All are likely to have some views relevant to the personal and social development of the young people and those views should be canvassed.

As a category, members of staff who do not work regularly in the establishment, and are therefore seen as external, may still play a highly significant role in the human environment. Therefore, many of the characteristics discussed are also important in their case. These include not only the obvious factors of specialisms and professional skills but also personalities and behaviour as models. Thus, they also require CRB clearance and should be aware of the aims and values of the setting so that, during their perhaps infrequent appearances, they do not inadvertently upset the residential programme.

Following very much the distinction between those staff who are part of the human environment and those who are external, the CRB offers different levels of check. The Enhanced Disclosure is required by all staff whose normal duties involve working in any way with the young people and, in particular, being in sole charge of young people under the age of 18. All others who work within the setting including administrative, domestic and ancillary staff require a Standard Disclosure. Apart from the CRB Disclosure, the recruitment procedures of the establishment should include the following:

- an identity check using an official document;
- two written references, both verified by direct contact;
- an interview;
- verification of any qualifications;
- the provision by the applicant of a full employment history which should be checked as far as possible by the establishment both with previous employers and with regard to any gaps. The details, together with issues of recruitment of staff from abroad are set out in a DfES Guidance Document (DfES/0278/2002) (2002).

One category of staff of particular relevance in the context of CRB checks is the Gap assistant, normally a young person from abroad, aged between 18 and the early twenties who provides support for residential staff. Such a person requires a 'certificate of good conduct' or equivalent but clearly great care needs to be taken, at least in the initial stages, about unsupervised access to the young people. Indeed, the National Minimum Standards for Boarding Schools (DoH, 2002e) lack clarity with regard to the detailed role of Gap assistants. It is therefore incumbent upon the school to provide a clear-cut job description (e.g. Holgate and Morgan, 2000).

Staff: dynamics

Interrelationships among the staff can have a profound influence upon the effectiveness and climate of the human environment. As with the young people, communications and the development of relationships are basic. In the case of staff, communications are likely to be far more wide-ranging from the informal through to the very formal. If the external members are included the modes of communication will be further increased.

The most important distinction is between the verbal and the written, and all communication of real consequence, particularly if there are likely to be further developments, should be recorded in writing. With the increasing use of personal computers and the development of a non-paper environment, this has become easier and quicker. Many establishments have specifically designed programmes for keeping the various forms of record. The other major development has been the use of the mobile telephone which means that staff on duty in various parts of the establishment can remain in communication with each other and the outside world. Indeed, it is very important, particularly in the larger settings, that mobile telephones are carried. Since a duty involves working with the young people in different parts of the establishment, external calls, possibly of importance, may be missed if there are only fixed telephones.

While there will be social and other relationships among members of staff, the most significant relationships are concerned with team work and leadership (Clough, 2000). To the young people, the staff team must appear consistent and fair in its approach. Whereas in a family the underpinning should be provided by affection, in a residential unit the foundation is closer to justice or fairness (Robinson, 1993). In counselling terms, there should be positive regard but affection may be seen as too strong a term.

Staff consistency is seen in planning and particularly in the implementation of policy. However, residential staff at whatever level are always in a position of potential role conflict (Callow, 1994). The expectations of their leaders or their team, the young people, the parents, the governors or management and possibly the public are usually not in accord. For example, in a boarding school parental interest may focus upon happiness, whereas house staff are looking at social development and the head at academic results. The governors are likely to be interested in all of these but in particular may have regard for safety and the fact that there is no adverse publicity. In a custodial setting, the desire of the public is basically for the removal of the young person from the streets and incarceration, the staff are interested in control and rehabilitation, the YJB is exercised about standards and the achievement of targets, and the parents are concerned primarily for the well-being of their offspring.

One issue which combines elements of all interests is risk (Burton, 1998). The risk factor is at the back of the minds of all parents or those with parental responsibility and it is not surprising that risk tends to be judged, in legal terms, in the light of the behaviour of a 'reasonable parent'. Most activities, from football to visiting the local shops, contain some element of risk. Taking into account the individuals involved, the key point for staff is to identify the likelihood of problems and, if necessary, to intervene. The possible effect of the occurrence of a specific hazard needs to be considered and a risk assessment made specific to the young people involved and to the level of staff control and guidance available. However, life itself involves risks and young people must learn to recognise and handle risk (Burton, 1993). It is only in the Standards for Care Homes for Young Adults that the importance of addressing risk as a preparation for life is a specific requirement.

Interaction between young people and staff

Interaction may be initiated by either the young people or the staff, or commonly it may be spontaneous from both sides. Staff and young people join together naturally in a variety of activities. However, there will always be a power differential in that the staff have overall responsibility for the welfare of the young people. Furthermore, although it is a teaching and learning environment for both staff and young people, fundamentally the staff are the teachers. One-sided interaction by staff may be characterised as staff intervention.

Intervention is one of the most sophisticated aspects of staff practice for staff who live and work with young people (Aguilera, 1994). In social work generally the term has been adopted as a specific procedure, normally concerned with families and children (Gupta and Coxhead, 1990). However, taken as a general term in the human environment, intervention occurs when staff influence young people to prevent or modify the result or course of events (Little and Mount, 1999). It could occur when senior staff feel the need to intervene in a situation which includes staff and young people but happens normally when staff take charge of a situation involving only young people. The subtlety comes in deciding when to intervene. When can the course of events be allowed to run and when does it appear that there is an unacceptable risk if there is no intervention? Is it more beneficial to allow things to happen the way they are? What is the effect of intervention? If young people are to learn through the experience of living together, is the intervention helpful? Other than in relatively obvious and extreme cases there are no rules about intervention. In cases of abuse or bullying, intervention is obvious and indeed a legal requirement, but what about in the event of a heated argument? In sport the referee or umpire intervenes to uphold the rules but in the normal living situation there are no such clear-cut guidelines. Some establishments have taken the parallel with football further and introduced the use of yellow and red cards for specified behaviours. If there is to be living and learning in the human environment, staff intervention will be necessary (Lishman, 1991).

Occasions when problems requiring intervention can be anticipated include:

- mealtimes;
- going to and getting up from bed;
- returning from a home visit;
- staff change-over time;
- group trips;
- lengthy unstructured periods of time;

- immediately prior to leaving the establishment;
- forthcoming court appearances or casework meetings (Kahan, 1994).

In the same volume, there is an inventory of signs that frequently presage trouble and a list of suggestions for the ways in which disorder or violence may be averted or ameliorated.

How is effective intervention learned? Some staff are more intuitive than others but expertise comes from experience, watching good practice by other members of staff and following a careful procedure of preview and review before and after events. Essentially, the requirement is for a very wide-ranging form of risk assessment, details of which are set out in relation to the physical environment.

Intervention also raises the question of discipline and control. Residence or boarding needs to be governed by rules and regulations, preferably the minimum number for the smooth operation of the establishment. Ideally the young people would have been involved in formulating the rules although in many settings this may not be practicable. It is however important that they understand the reasons for the rules and the necessity to abide by them. It is far easier to maintain a friendly, cooperative atmosphere if regulations are kept by consent rather than as a result of duress (Anderson, 1994b). There are specific guidelines to permissible controls and these are set out in Chapter 3.

Some rules govern what are essentially trivial pieces of behaviour such as lateness or talking after lights out, but, for the benefit of all, such rules need to be observed. At the other extreme there is behaviour which is illegal, in which case the police and other professionals should be involved. Other potential difficulties include the distinction between the individual and the group. Individual misbehaviour may be attributed relatively easily whereas that by a group may pose problems. It is likely that only certain members of the group were responsible and the punishment of the entire group would therefore be inappropriate if, perhaps at times, unavoidable. Furthermore, in investigating the issue, residential staff are likely to encounter group solidarity. Such 'street credibility' is, in most establishments, vital to the young people. However, it is through group silence that initiation rights, bullying and possibly abuse can survive.

Interaction is based upon communications and the development of relationships (Hargie et al., 1994). In the human environment verbal communications, talking and particularly listening, will predominate but the full scope will be used ranging from personal to impersonal, informal notes to public notices. Appropriate use of touch is also an important form of communication. Depending upon the location of the establishment on the family-to-formal continuum, ease of communication with individuals varies. For small groups, most contact can be at the personal level but for large groups there will need to be formal meetings. There is clearly a relationship between the size of the residential community and the regularity of meetings. In large communities, small units are likely to meet more regularly than the whole body. Indeed in many children's homes and small therapeutic units there are meetings at the start and at the end of each day to discuss the programme and its effect upon individuals. The smaller units also tend to meet informally more regularly. Those who share living space or a dormitory must meet several times a day. The higher the frequency of meetings, the more verbal communication is pre-eminent.

There is likely to be a positive correlation between the amount of verbal communication and the development of relationships. In the Occupational Standards for Staff (TOPSS UK Partnership, 2003), much is made of the skills of initiating, maintaining and ending relationships with the young people. This is the core of residential living and the focus of practice for the social pedagogue. The term 'social pedagogue' is widely recognised in continental Europe but in the UK is inadequately translated as residential worker or residential social worker. However, while there may be problems in agreement over the terminology, it is not difficult in practical terms to identify the group of professional workers who help other people by sharing substantially in their daily living (Courtioux et al., 1976).

According to the National Minimum Standards for the main types of setting, there should be a sound relationship between the staff and the young people. In the case of boarding schools (DoH, 2002e), this is the one Standard which can be considered pastoral, whereas for special boarding schools and children's homes the field of care is included in far more detail. Ideally, there would be a 'sound' or meaningful relationship between each member of staff and all the young people but, particularly in the larger units, this is unlikely to happen. At worst, there should be no obvious favouritism or discrimination. To initiate and sustain positive relationships requires some aspect, however small, of mutual 'chemistry' (Jacobs, 2000). At the other extreme, it is very important that relationships between individual members of staff and young people should not become too intense. Residence cannot and should not replicate the intensity of some relationships in family life (Robinson, 1994). Indeed, some young people come into residence to escape such intensities. Nonetheless, staff can still have a parenting role depending upon a number of factors including the emotional and chronological age of the young person, the family background and the known feelings of the parents. Indeed, it is suggested that there may be a verbal contract with parents agreeing on the needs of the young person (Kahan, 1994). Apart from some degree of empathy, staff also need to be aware that, for effective relationships, the power differential needs to be masked or temporarily reduced. If intervention is required, however, it is vital that there is a 'gap' between staff and young people and that staff can act with accepted authority.

The issue of affection or sympathy in relationships raises the question of touch. Since most physical and sexual abuse must involve touching, the subject is of particular significance. The danger is that the motives behind any touch may be misconstrued. There are no official guidelines available, and experience shows that the positive aspects of touch have been largely lost. Touch, in an appropriate manner and perceived as such by the young person, can be of great comfort. The subject is discussed in detail, with experiences from a variety of settings, by Cooke (1993), who advises that safety measures might include the following:

- ensure that any touch is public and is seen by others;
- know that the recipient is aware of the positive nature of the touch;
- make any embrace a sideways cuddle;
- record incidents, those initiated by a young person, in detail.

In a living and learning environment in which there is a high level of regard between the young people and the staff, the lack of touching, in certain circumstances such as grief, may be construed as abuse.

Within the human environment, staff facilitate activities, formal and informal, and use everyday occurrences to inculcate life skills which they can demonstrate. For such activities they make a continuous risk assessment so that, as far as possible, problems may be averted by early intervention. An example occurs when conflict resolution is addressed by the 'life-space interview' (Redl and Wineman, 1952). The young people in conflict are separated. Each provides an account of the event which led to the conflict and this is then contrasted with the account of the member of staff who was an observer of the occurrence. Mediation between these two views is then attempted. Such a procedure can be very effective in any setting but it depends crucially upon the observational capacity of the member of staff. Further, staff need to remember that their responses to the young people are subject to their own personal experiences and expectations. The requirement is to move from an accelerating to a decelerating environment (Davison, 1993). The goal of the staff member must be to reduce tensions and anxieties, and to achieve this the major component is time. If, in some way, a lull can be introduced into the events, tempers are likely to subside and, if the timing is correct, are unlikely to be regenerated. The reverse procedure is for a member of staff to encounter an inflammatory situation and to accelerate it by shouting, taking sides or making derogatory comments. A cooling-off period or in social work terminology, 'time out', can be highly beneficial not only for the individuals but also for the group.

Formal activities which represent interaction include all aspects of pastoral care and counselling, both with individuals and groups. However, it may be through informal activities that much of the effective pastoral work takes place. The essence of good practice is the informal chat. Although moving around the unit and talking to the young people does not appear to be effective work, for the thoughtful practitioner it provides the opportunity for real residential or boarding education. Leadership by staff (Hills and Child, 2000), both overt and particularly covert, can generate a vital and lively community. In contrast, a member of staff who merely goes through the routine, while watching as much television as possible, will do little to enhance living and learning and is likely to be unaware of antisocial behaviour. A proactive presence is the key to the interaction between young people and staff.

In the short term, the interaction provides the thread through daily living (Berry, 1975). In the longer term, such interactions assist the development of the young people and their various transitions from entry to leaving (Ainsworth and Fulcher, 1981). The external environment, in its entirety, and the physical environment enter the dynamic in providing opportunities but also imposing constraints. Although the dynamics between the young people are important particularly through peer group learning, it is the interaction between the young people and staff around which the main aspects of residential education revolve (O'Hagan, 2000).

Control

The core of the human environment, namely young people/staff interactions, is not isolated but its degree of insulation from normal life varies from sector to sector. Custodial, some psychiatric and some health settings are highly insulated whereas most children's homes, boarding schools, FE colleges and many special schools are very open. All are influenced by the physical environment and all to a certain degree by the external environment. There will be a clear distinction between urban and rural settings in the impact of the immediate neighbourhood and how it can be used by the human environment. However, the main determinant will remain the degree of enclosure of the establishment. For the young people, a secure setting in the middle of a city will seem little different from a similar setting in the countryside. The main aspect of the physical environment is the fabric, and an important consideration is whether or not it was purpose-built. Some establishments in almost all sectors were set up in large country houses. These required adaptation and have generally imposed some constraints upon the operation of the human environment. However, for a variety of reasons purpose-built accommodation can also impose constraints. With the costs of building, construction may not be of the highest quality and financial considerations favour minimisers or, at the most, sufficers rather than maximisers.

The degree to which the external environment impinges upon the human environment is crucial for a number of reasons. There appears to be a strong correlation between the success of an establishment in providing a secure, caring and stimulating *milieu* and its openness. The external environment also provides inputs to the young people/staff interaction system. Most significant are members of the family or those with parental responsibility and professionals who provide expertise which is not available among the full-time staff. These and others will be prominent in the interaction for limited periods but their influence may well last considerably longer. The external environment is also the major element in the overall control and management system which guides the operation of the human environment. The framework components – child protection, equal opportunities and legal issues – all represent external influences. The other controlling aspect is the value system of the establishment. The ultimate safeguard for this is the governing body or management team, which is strongly influenced by the external environment. There are controls at the internal, local, possibly regional and certainly national level. Examples would be, respectively: internal supervision, community support, regionally based inspections and National Minimum Standards. Therefore, however isolated or enclosed the establishment may appear, its barriers are penetrated by a variety of controlling inputs.

Outcome

Interactions in the human environment generate the developmental components, are controlled by the framework components and vary according to the time components. Therefore, the resultant is the output of the entire residential system of the establishment. However, while the other sets of components obtain everywhere, the importance of each developmental component varies according to the type of establishment. For instance, custodial, psychiatric and military together with some health settings, special schools, boarding schools and FE colleges have health, education and care elements within the establishment. Some health settings have only health and care while education is external. Some boarding schools and therapeutic communities have only education and care, with health being external. Children's homes, boarding school hostels, some FE colleges and refugee centres are likely to have only care on the premises with both education and health external (Figure 2.5). Thus, the only common component is care, the fundamental basis of residence. With this constraint in mind, the main output is the product of residential or boarding education demonstrated in the lives of the young people who have been through the system.

Other outputs include the ambience of the establishment and, it is hoped, a progression in good practice by staff. Beyond these, there are many less tangible outputs such as the influence on society of the young people. Many of these factors and ideas for their evaluation were discussed in Anderson and King (1994). As a result of work, in a variety of settings, the key components for assessment were identified as: (1) structure, (2) interrelationships, (3) characteristics, (4) ambience. Structure refers to the aspects of supervision, control, routine and flexibility producing the social framework for the interrelationships. The output of the interrelationships between all of those involved in the operation of the establishment is the community life. At any one time, the results of community life may be judged by the characteristics common to the behaviour of the young people. The ambience refers to the overall feel (Kahan, 1994) of the community. This can only be evaluated after a reasonable period of acquaintance. If the characteristics or ambience do not accord with the aims and values of the establishment, then changes can be made to the sub-systems. This is only, of course,

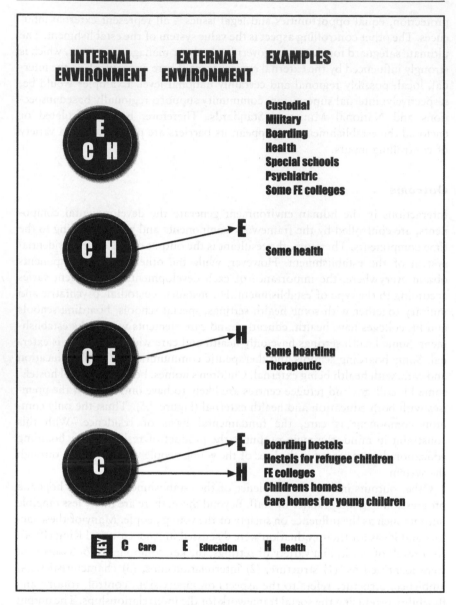

Figure 2.5   Environment and type of setting

possible if those sub-systems have been identified and analysed, and the workings of the establishment are no longer viewed as merely a black box.

Physical environment

The physical environment (Anderson and King, 1994) not only provides a framework for the human environment but also insulates it from the external environment. The human environment, with some additions from the external environment, and the physical environment mutually affect each other in that, for example, the physical environment imposes limits on activities which may need to be altered. At the same time, the physical environment is likely to be modified to take account of certain activities.

From the viewpoint of the young people and staff, the physical environment is significant for a number of reasons. Like any boundary, it defines the limits of the establishment (either the edge of the grounds or the buildings) and provides a barrier to the world outside. Thereby, it should ensure safety for the young people, a constant in any broadly based risk assessment. Indeed, the risk assessment of the physical environment as opposed to either the human or the external environment is relatively more predictable. The barrier is, however, porous in that its second function is as a control. It should provide controlled entry to the establishment and sub-units within the establishment. In general, the public will be prohibited from entering the grounds, the entry of people from the external environment will be closely monitored and, within the buildings, there will be rooms which are entirely private. The level of control will define the openness of the establishment, an issue not only of physical but also of psychological importance.

As a result of these boundary functions, the physical environment should provide the foundation for security. The young people should feel not only safe from immediate danger but also psychologically protected and untroubled so that they can benefit from the residential experience. This is particularly important for damaged young people who need to feel not only free from the threat of abuse but also integrated into a caring community. The physical environment can also operate to keep the young people inside. Absconding can occur from any residential setting but the more obvious examples of this particular function occur with custodial care, psychiatric units and some special schools and homes (Safe on the Streets Research Team, 1999).

It is in the context of the physical environment that there is the most clearly defined framework within which staff should conduct a risk assessment. There are basically four aspects requiring such assessment:

1   The buildings, furnishings and equipment.
2   The services.
3   The grounds, and particularly the play areas used.

4   Parts of the local area external to the settings which are most frequented by the young people.

In each case there are four stages in the procedure, details of which need to be recorded:

1   Make a detailed inspection and note all the possible hazards, including those resulting from damage or wear and tear.
2   For each hazard noted, write down the potential for accident or harm to the young people during the course of carrying out their normal activities.
3   Decide on the action to be taken to minimise or eliminate the possible effect of the hazard. Record your decision and inform the necessary authorities so that action may be taken as quickly as possible.
4   Monitor the situation and check that the risk has been minimised or eliminated as appropriate.

Before making the risk assessment, it is important to have inspected earlier such assessments to ascertain that action has been taken about previous hazards identified. However, it must be realised that, despite every effort by staff, a risk-free environment cannot be produced. Indeed, where people are living together in groups it is doubtful whether such a situation exists let alone whether it would be wholly desirable.

Such a procedure is a more formalised example of the preview which residential staff should undertake before overseeing any activities with the young people. Rather than concerns about the fabric of the establishment, the risk may involve mixing particular young people together, contravening some aspect of the law, allowing the entry of a particular visitor or initiating some form of activity. The risk must be assessed against any potential benefits and the staff member should act as a responsible parent.

The physical environment enhances some activities, for example, through the possession of a football pitch, but may constrain others, for example, where the educational provision is located in the external environment. Through the divisions of space, the physical environment offers community and individual development with larger common rooms and smaller individual rooms. The division of space and many other aspects of the physical environment provide a strong indication of the value system of the establishment particularly whether it tends towards participative or authoritarian. This may be shown not only by room size and distribution but also by control of access, quality and style of décor and communications of all types. For the young people, the physical environment is likely to be closely associated with home. In this, there may be some difference between those who board and those whose period of residence is continuous. However, in all cases, there should be a private bed space with some furnishing which is also considered private, even if it only amounts to a drawer.

Personal space, which may be a separate room, a shared room or part of a dormitory or, in some cases, one tier of a bunk-bed, is an emotive issue. Residential living involves commitment in that, whether they wished it or not, the young people show complete commitment by sleeping in the establishment. It is recognised psychologically that at rest a person is at his or her most vulnerable, and therefore the bed is the core of an individual's personal space. This issue is considered sufficiently significant to be covered in the guidance to the *Children Act* (DoH, 1991e). Within reason, young people should be permitted to have an array of their own possessions and decorations so that they feel at home. Clearly, if those impedimenta cause offence to others or protrude into a neighbouring personal space, some control is necessary (FitzGerald, 1994).

A common problem is the subject matter of posters, and a reasonable rule would seem to be that they should be removed if cleaners or others who need to work in the space are caused offence. Another concern is that of personal keys and lockable doors and drawers. If the door of a room can be locked by the occupant, this shows that privacy is taken seriously. On the other hand, locked doors are hardly in the spirit of residential community living and undoubtedly represent a safety hazard. These points may be argued either way but one vital condition should be that before opening a door to a private room, any visitor, whether staff or young person, should knock. In all settings, there is a general rule that nobody enters a private room without permission.

The physical environment also contributes to, and in some cases dominates, the ambience of the establishment. Despite, in many cases, a thoughtful design by architects, it is very difficult in custodial settings to escape the view of high walls. If a school is in a large old country house, the environment requires modification to make it homely. In health settings, great efforts are made to decorate hospital wards so that they appear less institutional.

These functions raise a number of dichotomies, between each of which a balance needs to be struck. Access should be encouraged to ensure an open society and all the benefits of external influences but there also needs to be safety and security. Within the buildings, community living and residential education should predominate but public events must be judged against the value of privacy. Ideally the young people make progress towards independence and should therefore have as much freedom of choice as possible, but in the interests of all there must be control and surveillance. Rights and fulfilment must be safeguarded but not at the expense of another young person's rights or fulfilment. To manage the establishment, there has to be a staff hierarchy but activities should be arranged, as far as is reasonable, to focus upon equality and a participative approach.

Built environment

The built environment (Anderson and King, 1994) is a subject of study in its own right and its importance has been increasingly realised. *Care and*

Treatment in a Planned Environment (Department of Health and Social Security, 1972) was a landmark publication but since then there have been a number of government reports which have included a focus on the fabric, notably *Homes are for Living In* (DoH, 1989a). The relationship of the built to the physical environment is of interest, particularly when concerns over security are raised. For example, in boarding settings the built environment is commonly located some distance from the boundary, the limit of the physical environment. This disposition contrasts sharply with that found in some other setting types, notably custodial care (Figure 2.6). In secure settings there will be no generally accessible physical environment beyond the built environment boundary (Blumenthal, 1985).

The first impression for the young people about to be resident is likely to be scale. Many of the buildings may be large and will appear particularly sizeable to children aged 11 or 12. The apparently vast scale of the built environment seems to reduce with familiarity and increasing progress through adolescence. Some of the buildings, for reasons of security, appear forbidding. In contrast, some of the smaller units are accommodated in normal housing. Children's homes and some special schools may occupy domestic buildings in local housing estates. It must be realised that the imposing buildings and those which are dominated by considerations of security both militate against ease of induction. The thoughts of a small child going from a primary school of 100 children

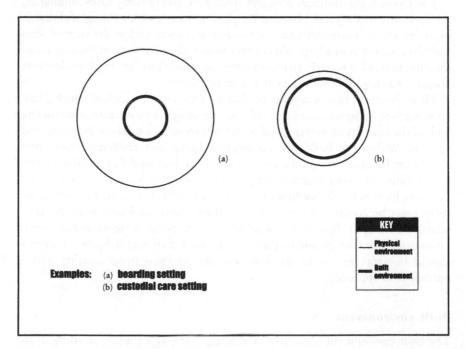

Figure 2.6   Location of the built environments

to a boarding school of 650 can only be imagined. It is no wonder that, for all, the rite of passage takes some while to complete and, for some, it may remain incomplete.

According to Geddes and Gutman (1977), the following properties of the built environment are of significance with regard to behaviour:

- spatial organisation: the relative location of the various facilities;
- circulation systems: the spaces for the movement of people;
- communication systems: aspects which provide information and ideas for the residence, including windows, pictures, telephones and notices;
- ambient properties: these include illumination, heating, ventilation, humidity and noise levels;
- visual properties: the perceived appearance of the environment including colour, style, cleanliness and degree of vandalism;
- amenities: these are related to specific social activities and include kitchens, bedrooms and bathrooms;
- symbolic factors: these indicate social values such as equality or hierarchy;
- architectonic properties: these are the large-scale aesthetic qualities.

At another level, the built environment may be divided into a number of areas according to function:

- domestic;
- administrative;
- shared;
- personal or private.

(Anderson and King, 1994).

In some settings there will also be specialised rooms such as surgeries or those housing medical facilities, 'time-out' rooms or therapy units.

As discussed in Porteous (1977), the built environment may also be seen in terms of territoriality and the distinction between the home base and the home range, the area outside the establishment which is used particularly by the young people. Within the home base, there will be several patterns of usage of the various facilities and these may in time produce changes in the built environment. One example would be activity centres, the areas in which informal meetings and activities commonly occur. Where is the best place for staff to enjoy a leisure-time chat with the young people? This may be a common room but is equally likely to be a kitchen or even a drying room.

Surroundings

Apart from the built environment the other elements of the physical environment range from the grounds (Department for Education and Employment

(DfEE), 1997) and other external spaces to the local community and the areas outside the perimeter of the setting which are used regularly by the young people. In custodial care, the grounds of any significance are all internal to the boundary and even the line of the built environment. In boarding schools, the local community may play a relatively large role in the life of the school. For example, there may be shared sporting and cultural activities together with community service. Grounds can clearly be used for a wide range of leisure activities, for various forms of work experience and for teaching, but their use is governed very much by the type of setting. The major direct educational use of grounds probably occurs in FE colleges in which horticulture and aspects of agriculture are studied. Elsewhere, if access is allowed, grounds may have utilitarian as well as aesthetic value. In general terms, grounds have particular value for boarding schools, some special schools and FE colleges together with some children's homes and health settings. For many health settings, children's homes and custodial care units, the grounds outside the built environment may be of limited utility.

In making an assessment in parallel to that made for the human environment, the overall situation, including the regional attributes and the local community and the actual site and the area immediately adjacent to the buildings, require consideration. Within the built environment itself form and function and the relationship between the two is of importance. Development may be seen in alterations in the physical environment as the establishment changes. The overall 'feel' of the physical fabric and its surroundings, analogous to the ambience of the human environment, may be categorised as the '*milieu*' (Anderson and King, 1994).

External environment

The overriding factor of importance is the degree to which the external environment is able to penetrate the human environment of the establishment. The key component of the external environment is the family or those with delegated parental responsibility, and the more open the setting, the greater the chance of partnership to support the development of the young people. Clearly there needs to be a balance between openness and security and, for secure settings, openness has to be a secondary consideration. There will be some external influences, such as those concerned with the law, for all establishments. However, the full array of benefits which may result from close cooperation with the external environment will be reduced according to the degree of enclosure. Among the types of setting, boarding schools and FE colleges are likely to be the most open while custodial and psychiatric settings will be predominantly closed. Indeed, visits from family members may need to be tightly controlled.

The external environment provides safeguards. An example is the Area Child Protection Committee (ACPC), shortly to be replaced by the Local

Safeguarding Children Board (Green Paper, 2003), which will coordinate the functions of all partner agencies in relation to the welfare of young people. It is envisaged that there will be a Director of Children's Services for each local authority. The Director will be accountable for Social Services, education and all services for young people delegated to the local authority by other services. In most authorities this will result in a Children's Department with responsibility for all young people in its area. Support for young people will also be provided by a lead council member specially designated to be responsible for children's welfare. Furthermore, it is envisaged that there will eventually be Children's Trusts which would incorporate educational, social and health functions and may also include Connexions and Youth Offending Teams (YOTs). The safeguards at national level will continue to comprise standard-setting mechanisms and an integrated inspection framework. All settings, whether open or closed, will need to work with these various agencies. The governors or managers of the establishment also provide statutory safeguards for the young people.

Apart from safeguards generally, the external environment is a source of advice, consultancy, inspection, services, action and friendship. Any or all of the following may be involved: health visitors, general practitioners, social workers, education welfare officers, youth and community workers, Connexions, personal advisers, educational psychologists, children's mental health professionals, speech and language therapists and other allied health professionals, young people's substance misuse workers, learning mentors and school support staff, school nurses and possibly home visitors, volunteers and mentors and statutory and voluntary homelessness agencies. All must be checked by the CRB.

Some of these professionals have a right of entry, others come by invitation. For the latter, it is important to develop a network of carefully selected individuals who understand the values, ethos and aims of the setting. Some will come on occasional visits, sometimes unannounced, others will be regular visitors working as part of the staff team. Non-professionals may offer a range of services, religious, cultural and sporting. They may, as with those representing organisations such as Voice of the Child in Care, appear only for the purpose of offering friendship to the young people. It is vital that in any residential setting, the young people have access to a responsible adult in the external environment upon whom they can call if they have serious problems. The general term for such people is 'independent visitor' and their functions may include visiting, advising, befriending, representation and possibly advocacy. In addition, for young people in the Youth Justice System there are YOTs and probation services (Crimmens and Pitts, 2000).

The most significant element of the external environment is the family (Chakrabarti and Hill, 2000) or those with parental responsibility, and their relationship with the young people is vital. The improvement of parenting is a key element in government policy with regard to both families and young people. A fundamental issue is that the number of characteristics which distinguish the family unit is continually diminishing. Some parents are married and live together, others live apart; some parents are unmarried and live together and some live apart. Second and subsequent marriages can result in an array of step- and half-relationships. Single-parent families, usually parented by the mother, are common. Some families are nuclear, others are extended. It must be increasingly difficult for young people to make sense of their backgrounds. The traditional concept of the family as a unit which is stable in the long term, with its own support network, has been severely eroded. Current lifestyles and increasing mobility mean that few families have relatives living nearby on whom they can rely.

There are many other questions that may be asked on the subject, but particularly relevant queries concern the functioning of the family. Can it be described as functional or dysfunctional? In the major biological functions of procreation and nurturing, the nurturing appears to be increasingly neglected (Winnicott, 1957). Parenting is now included under various headings in the curriculum of schools and can therefore influence young people in residential and boarding education and care. Nonetheless, biological ties are extremely resilient and all settings seek relationships with families so that there can be at least an element of shared decision making. In boarding schools, this is seen as a partnership, although, in some cases, this may be a somewhat Utopian view. Certainly if there is weekly boarding, it would appear more realistic. In other settings, for various reasons, the partnership tends to be weaker. In hospital schools and special schools concerned with health problems, much of the decision making is beyond the expertise of most families but certainly they should be fully consulted. For education and personal development, their views must be sought. Many young people are in social settings as a result of family problems and therefore response from families is likely to be limited. In custodial care, family input may have been deviant and contact with the young people has to be carefully regulated. As the relationship varies according to type of establishment so does family support. However, it is legally incumbent upon the establishment to keep families informed of decisions which affect the young people and it is important to ensure a reasonable regime of visits.

Apart from safeguards, it is also through the external environment that valid assessment of the establishment can be made. This is not to say that internal assessment is invalid but that it is unlikely to carry the weight and universal regard of something made externally and possibly nationally. Ideally, internal and external measures would both be used. Certainly, the aim for the National Minimum Standards is that the best possible conditions obtain inside. The production of League Tables for academic achievement is a relatively crude procedure but it has a certain national validity, although when examined in detail, there are many objections which could be raised. However, compared with the evaluation of personal and social development, academic progress is relatively easy to measure.

The assessment of the effectiveness of residential and boarding establishments can never be definitive. There are many variables and few controls. Even more difficult for researchers is the isolation of residence or boarding itself as a factor. Most of the evidence is likely to be qualitative and resistant to standard validation procedures. Nonetheless, it should be possible to obtain a general overview which is scientifically acceptable. If, through theoretical, evaluative and empirical action research, it is possible to establish measures for the effectiveness of residential settings, then improved matching with the young people becomes a reality. The DoH (1998b) has a range of projects including Quality Protects and Choice Protects in which routes into care are examined and evaluated, but the accent is very much upon foster care and the only type of setting normally considered is the children's home. The field of external evaluation, standards and inspections is now receiving serious attention and has become a key factor in the external environment for all settings.

Chapter 3

Framework components

The framework components, which in the model surround the environmental components, provide the boundaries for the operation of the establishment. Any setting for young people requires some form of legal control, and the *Children Act* (1989) established the basis for all sectors other than custodial care and military training establishments. Young people in custodial care have now been brought under the *Children Act* (1989) and the fact that those under the age of 18 were removed from active duty before the invasion of Iraq (2003) indicated that, in terms of child protection, military personnel are also receiving serious attention. According to their status, whether maintained, non-maintained or independent, residential and boarding establishments for young people have varying degrees of autonomy. However, the *Children Act* (1989) and subsequent legislation has set out the limits very clearly. Most legal components are based upon the *United Nations Convention on the Rights of the Child* (1987) which was ratified by the UK in 1991. Thus all young people below the age of 18 are effectively under international law and national law together with regional and local regulations and in-house rules and guidelines. Three terms are of general relevance:

1   Acts are Acts of Parliament which are laws of the land by which everybody is bound.
2   Regulations are secondary legislations, but are similarly binding.
3   Guidance is not itself legislation but constitutes a statement of good practice.

For convenience, the law relating to residential and boarding education and care may be subdivided into relevant elements:

•   child protection;
•   duties and responsibilities, principally of residential staff;
•   human rights and, in particular, non-discrimination;
•   factors related to residence.

The focus of legislation for young people is upon protection from harm. This is concerned not only with negatives but is also about defining the basic rights and needs of young people. Human rights legislation covers a wide variety of topics but it is significant that in the *Convention on the Rights of the Child* Article No. 2 is entitled *Right to Non-Discrimination.* In any residential setting, this must be a fundamental aim which underpins all activities. Law relating to the staff in residential environments covers legal responsibilities, duty of care and a range of issues involving support for the young people (Franklin, 2002). Acts of Parliament of particular importance in the residential setting include the *Fire Precautions Act* (1971), the *Health and Safety at Work Act* (1974) and the *Food Safety Act* (1990), together with legislation on employment, vehicles and planning.

Human rights and factors related to residence range widely in their coverage, and therefore vary in their detailed application according to the setting and particularly the sector. Child protection and equal opportunities or non-discrimination are in contrast universal requirements covering the fundamental rights of the young people. Therefore, while all legal aspects contribute to the framework, an appropriate summary is provided by three: child protection, equal opportunities and legal issues, which is taken to cover all the remaining aspects of the law.

There are many other points about the law which are of importance for the living and learning environment, one of which is its relative malleability. For residence, some aspects of the law are clear-cut and brook no argument. An example is the age for consuming alcohol. The establishment must operate within the law of the land and cannot afford to turn a blind eye to its transgression. Other aspects are less clearly defined in that there is some room for interpretation and discussion. The duty of care, or *in loco parentis,* element would fall into this category. Furthermore, for residential living, some parts of the law are suggestive without being prescriptive (Brayne and Martin, 1999).

For the model, the legal framework components, taken to occupy three sides of the boundary, are all, of course, imposed from outside and are therefore part of the external environment. The fourth side is the internally generated constraint which may be characterised as philosophy/aims/ethos (Figure 3.1). This subsumes the ideas and concepts which provide the driving force for the establishment. At a daily level they are seen in procedures, policies, rules and regulations which address proximate aims. For most settings, the philosophy written or unwritten, voiced or unvoiced, extends beyond the proximate. The philosophy provides the foundation for all the developmental components for the young people. It is part of the framework since the human environment is constrained from activities which contravene the ethos. The relationship between the components is that the law, firmly yoked to philosophy/aims/ethos, informs and governs the environmental components which themselves generate the developmental components (Figure 3.2). However, the philosophy is different from the remaining three because it is self-imposed and there are no direct

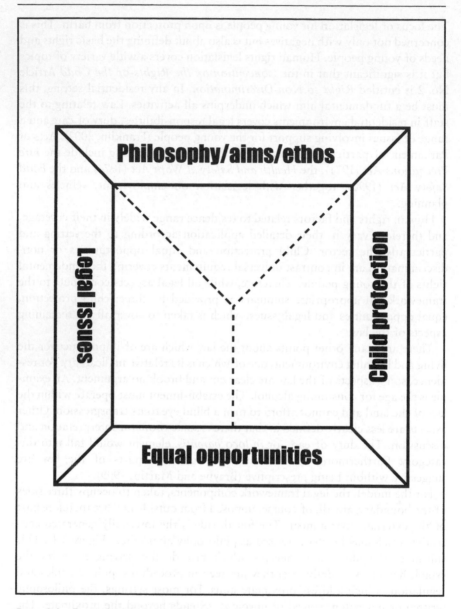

Philosophy/aims/ethos

Legal issues

Child protection

Equal opportunities

Figure 3.1 Framework components

legal constraints involved. Furthermore, elements of the philosophy, and particularly its application, may change over time rather more obviously and frequently than sections of the law.

The philosophy of most establishments is rooted in a number of basic aims covering broadly: child welfare, realisation of potential and preparation for the

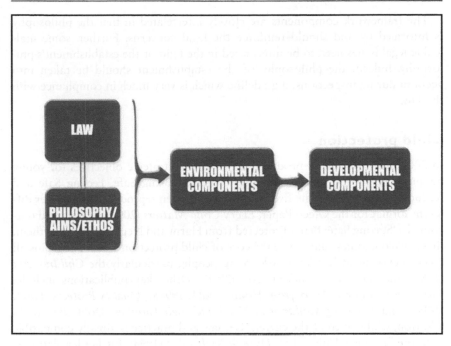

Figure 3.2   Relationship between philosophy and law

future. These points are likely to be set out in any statement of principles or mission statement. The main variation will involve how these are defined and how they are to be achieved. What exactly constitutes welfare? What exactly do we mean by the future? Realisation of potential raises problems in that for any one individual it is almost impossible to interpret while its evaluation produces almost insuperable difficulties. It might be questioned whether anybody realises his or her potential. Even if the potential could be defined, its realisation may only become apparent in an obituary.

With regard to philosophy, one great advantage which the boarding schools share with few other settings is tradition. Some hospitals are obviously long established and certain children's homes, therapeutic communities and special schools have been running for a sufficiently long time to have accumulated some tradition. Having developed an ethos over a long period of time gives the internal constraint a particular strength. For older settings, a particularly pervasive factor is the religious tradition with its accent on strong moral values. There may be links with the original form of residential life, the monastic tradition, which still has much to offer as a model (Jack, 1998). For newer establishments, the philosophy tends to be guided by the ideas of the current manager or principal. As with so many things in residence, there needs to be a balance between sustaining tradition and remaining sufficiently flexible that relevant changes in society may be accommodated.

The framework components are closely interrelated in that the philosophy is informed by and should reinforce the legal concerns. Further, some malleable legal issues need to be interpreted in the light of the establishment's philosophy. Indeed, the philosophy of the establishment should be taken into account during inspections, a guideline which is very much in compliance with the law.

Child protection

In 2003, the government produced a list of five strategic objectives for young people. The second objective is: 'Staying Safe: Being Safe, Feeling Safe and Reducing Risks'. The same five objectives have been reproduced in a rather different format for the Green Paper, *Every Child Matters* (2003). The second outcome is: 'Staying Safe: Being Protected from Harm and Neglect'. Between them, these two outcomes summarise the core of child protection which underpins all recent government legislation on young people, particularly the *Children Act* (1989) and the *Care Standards Act* (2000). Other key publications include: *Caring for Children Away from Home* (DoH, 1998a), *Quality Protects* (DoH, 1998b) and *Assessing Children in Need and their Families* (DoH, 2000a). In addition, while much of the current UK law and practice is already compatible with the European Union (EU) *Human Rights Act* (1998), further legislation is being enacted to bring the country totally into line.

Although the term 'child protection' is generally taken to refer to some recognisable form of abuse, the range of legislation illustrates the point that it has a far broader application. This is set out clearly in the *Children Act* (1989) in which the legal definition of child abuse is given as:

> the primary justification for the state to initiate proceedings seeking compulsory powers is actual or likely harm to the child, where harm includes both ill-treatment (which includes sexual abuse and non-physical ill-treatment such as emotional abuse) and the impairment of health for development, health meaning physical or mental health, and development meaning physical, intellectual, emotional, social or behavioural development.

Child protection may therefore be taken to cover all aspects of life in residential and boarding education and care, particularly the developmental components. Further evidence for this assertion is drawn from the *Care Standards Act* (2000), in that National Minimum Standards have been published:

> to determine whether it (residential establishment) is complying with its legal obligation to safeguard and promote the welfare of children and young people.

In all settings where Standards obtain, assessment is focused upon policies, premises and people. Assessment is obviously crucial for the specific procedures connected with abuse but also for complaints procedures, for staff selection and for staff training. It impacts on all activities in that each demands a preview and a review together with some form of risk assessment. This raises another issue relevant to all forms of residential education and care: what is an acceptable risk? In many ways, life is made up of risks and, for life after residence and independence, it is important that the young people have an opportunity to take risks. Acceptable risk is best seen as one which, in the circumstances, would be taken by a careful parent. Reasonable supervision is to be expected but the interpretation of this varies according to the sector and setting. For example, if a boarding school is compared with a special school for young people with behavioural, emotional and social development difficulties, the staff ratio will be considerably lower in the former and staff presence will be conspicuously less.

Abuse, depending upon its definition, can merge with bullying (DfE, 1994), aspects of discrimination and other forms of indiscipline. All involve protection from harm. Within the field of harm, abuse must be the focus since among all the risks, certain forms of abuse are probably the most likely to have extreme long-term effects. Such abuse may be physical, emotional or sexual (Davis, 1993; Farmer and Pollock, 1998) but it can also come about through neglect or through the operation of the institution itself (Stanley *et al.*, 1999). A valuable discussion on child protection in the residential care system is provided by The Violence Against Children Study Group (1999). Clearly the basic definitions relating to these terms, together with the warning signs for each, must be familiar to the residential staff and all other members of the staff who commonly come into contact with the young people. All staff must also know the procedure should they become aware of abuse, or alleged abuse, through observation, disclosure or any other means. Each establishment should have a designated officer whose identity is known to all members of staff. The designated officer works closely with the ACPC (DoH *et al.*, 1999), to be renamed the Local Safeguarding Children Board (LSCB). Apart from a knowledge of what happens when abuse is alleged, staff must be well acquainted with all aspects of confidentiality as set out in the *Data Protection Act* (1998). Since the subject raises so many issues related to all aspects of residential living, child protection is the key training requirement for all staff who work directly with the young people (Casson and Manning, 1997).

The basic safeguards for all young people living away from home are set out in detail in *Working Together to Safeguard Children* (DoH *et al.*, 1999), and include the following:

• children feel valued and respected;
• the residential establishment is open to the external world;

- staff are trained in all aspects of safeguarding children, are alert to the vulnerabilities of risks and harm and are knowledgeable about the implementation of child protection procedures;
- children have access to a trusted adult outside the establishment and should be aware of external services available including ChildLine;
- there should be an effective and readily accessible complaints procedure and a complaints register;
- staff recruitment and selection procedures are rigorous;
- there are clear procedures and support systems, including guarantees to 'whistle blowers', in place for dealing with expressions of concern by staff about other staff;
- there is respect for diversity and a clear equal opportunities policy;
- effective staff supervision and support is required for all staff, including administrative, maintenance, temporary staff and volunteers;
- staff are alert to the risks for children in the external environment, including with their families.

The volume sets out the entire procedure for inter-agency working to safeguard and promote the welfare of children, and includes sections on roles and responsibilities, ACPCs, handling individual cases, and child protection in specific circumstances. A complementary work (London Child Protection Committee, n.d.) provides an update and sets out a very full list of child protection issues in specific circumstances:

- child pornography and the internet;
- racial and religious harassment;
- forced marriage of a child;
- families where a parent is involved in prostitution;
- disabled children;
- families where a parent has learning difficulties;
- parents who misuse drugs or alcohol;
- enduring and/or severe parental mental illness;
- young carers;
- self-harming and suicidal behaviour;
- pregnancy of child;
- looked after children and others living away from home;
- foreign exchange visits;
- surrogacy;
- begging.

There are also important sections on children in whom illness is fabricated or induced, female genital mutilation, abuse by children, missing children, children involved in prostitution, children trafficking and exploitation, and unexplained death of a child. These various lists provide a full picture of the scope of child protection and, although in any one setting most of the circumstances are unlikely to be encountered, the range of issues needs to be appreciated by residential staff.

Legal issues

Apart from legislation concerning child protection and non-discrimination, several other sectors of the law apply wholly or partially to residential child care. Indeed, a distinction might be made between general law which everybody must follow and law which is specific to residential life. This does not mean that residential staff have to be trained in the law but that they need to have some overall idea of what is covered, and in particular where to find any relevant legislation. This implies, in particular, familiarity with the *Children Act* (1989), but also a more detailed knowledge of legal aspects of their own practice particularly with regard to child protection, duty of care and non-discrimination.

For staff, relevant law with the related policies and procedures of the establishment may be considered at three levels:

1   That which is directly related to the young people.
2   That which concerns the organisation and operation of the establishment.
3   That concerned predominantly with management.

All staff would benefit from an overview of all three levels but, for detailed and even definitive knowledge, there is a reduction in the 'need to know factor' from the first to the last.

The *Children Act* (1989), the *Human Rights Act* (1998) (in force from 1 October 2000), and the *Care Standards Act* (2000) (in force from 1 April 2002) provide the main elements of the framework within which residential staff work and manage young people. The staff have, effectively, a parenting role but they are not and must never see themselves as surrogate parents. Their position *in loco parentis* is geographical rather than legal.

The *Care Standards Act* (2000) has brought into law amendments to the *Children Act* (1989) while changes attendant upon the *Human Rights Act* (1998) are still in train. For life in the human environment, the main caring duties set out in the various Acts cover:

- pastoral care;
- discipline;
- health and medical concerns;
- child protection and safety generally;
- confidentiality;
- data protection.

In the external environment the Acts deal with two areas of particular importance:

1   Relationships with those with parental responsibility.
2   Responsibility for the young people in both civil law and criminal law.

Related duties include the need to establish a complaints procedure and to carry out risk assessment.

Young people have the right to complain about any aspect of the establishment. The main element in the procedure is that there are clear communication lines which the young people are encouraged to use and which cover both designated internal carers and appropriate external agents. In addition, there should be confidential links with independent visitors. There must also, of course, be channels for staff complaints.

Apart from these aspects of the law, there is legal compliance concerned with the general field of health and safety, including fire, hygiene, food, noise, electricity and first aid (Stock, 1993). Related to it are legal rights at various ages and this is another area with which all staff should be conversant. The ages at which young people can lawfully carry out certain acts vary and there is a set inventory for ages 13, 14, 15, 16, 17 and 18 (Boyd, 1999).

The range of law related to young people living away from home in groups is wide. All settings live within the law of the land and all are controlled by laws concerning young people. The *Children Act* (1989) has now been brought to bear on young people in custodial care but still does not cover young people in military training or refugee centres. According to the type of residence, certain aspects of the law will be more or less important. The legal implications of recreational and educational visits away from the establishment will be of great importance in boarding schools but considerably less significant in many health settings and secure units. Other examples showing variations in application include personal searches, several legal aspects of health, links to those with parental responsibility and freedom of association between young people.

The Children Act (1989)

This Act has been described as the most comprehensive piece of legislation which Parliament has ever enacted about young people (Allen, 1992). It provides a new framework for the care and upbringing of all young people, and in so doing strikes a new balance between family autonomy and the protection of young people. The provisions are based upon principles which apply to all young people so that all are treated in the same way before the law. Within the Act there are three foci:

1   Child welfare.
2   Parental responsibility.
3   Decision making involving children (Willow, 1996).

The Act is supported by eleven volumes of regulations and guidance and, of these, the introduction together with volumes 4, 5, 6 and 7 are of particular importance for residential staff and those with managerial responsibility. The introduction includes definitions and provides a general coverage of children who are looked after by local authorities, and the welfare of children away from home. Volume 4 sets out the care of children living away from home in depth and, despite the fact that the focus is children's homes, it well repays consideration by all staff involved in residential and boarding education and care. Volume 5 deals with independent schools and volume 6 children with disabilities. The section specifically on residential care for children with disabilities includes subsections on: children accommodated in residential care, nursing and mental nursing homes; in secure accommodation; by health or education authorities; and in independent schools. Volume 7 is concerned with guardians *ad litem* but does include details on other, court-related issues. The eleven volumes are supported by a further range of publications (e.g. *The Welfare of Children in Boarding Schools: Practice Guide* (DoH, 1991a, 1991b, 1991c, 1991d, 1991e)).

The philosophy underpinning the Act is that, while the first duty is to promote and safeguard the young person's welfare, the best place for the young person to be brought up is usually in his/her own family. While there may be fundamental agreement with this statement, it does raise a number of obvious issues for residential and boarding education and care. Young people live away from home in some settings as a result of choice, in others through referral. What are the compensations for extra-familial living? Broadly speaking, in secure accommodation and much of the health and social provision, the decision is reached, assuming it is not mandatory, that it is in the best interests of the young person to live away from the family. The length of time involved will vary according to the specific case and the treatment prescribed. In some cases, those with parental responsibility need to acquiesce in the decision but in many, there are statutory controls. In the case of special schools there is more choice, in that for many young people there could be equivalent day care provision available. However, there may be boarding need through parental absence abroad, mobility or family problems of various kinds. For young people in the military, the choice is essentially about joining the military rather than about selecting any particular training base. In FE colleges, residence in many cases reflects boarding need through the distance of the college from the home of the young person. This occurs particularly when the choice of course is one which is not generally available throughout FE colleges. Colleges with particular specialisation may provide on-site accommodation or support young people under the age of 18 in selecting lodgings. Some young people in FE accommodation undoubtedly want to live away from their families.

Boarding schools and FE colleges are in general the most open of all the settings and can therefore develop the closest relationship with families or those with parental responsibility. This point clearly applies less, if at all, to young people coming to UK boarding schools from abroad and also to those who live a long distance from the school. Weekly boarding is an attempt to obtain the best of residence and the best of home life.

It must also be remembered that there have been several government reports, most notably the Martin Report (1960), which identified a range of boarding needs. Types of need, for which the LEA should consider support, were defined in the following terms:

- when both parents were abroad;
- when parents are in this country but liable to frequent moves due to their occupation;
- when the home circumstances are seriously prejudicial to the normal development of the child;
- when the child has a special aptitude requiring training which can only be given by a boarding education.

In practice, with the exceptions of music and ballet, the fourth category has not loomed large in decision making. Broadly speaking, those young people with boarding need either lack a permanent home sufficiently near a school or have family problems. Details of the Martin Report and its application are set out in Lambert (1966). In the most recent survey to examine residential and boarding education and care (Anderson and Morgan, 1987), some two-thirds of pupils in maintained boarding schools and up to 50 per cent in many independent schools came within these two categories. There remain many young people – it is surmised well over half the population of many of the larger boarding schools – who are in boarding because it is deemed to be beneficial for them. Certainly, given the pace of life and the lifestyle of many families today, the advantages of boarding for social development can be seen. There remains in the UK a tradition of sending young people to boarding school but this is declining and it is now normal in many schools for the majority of residents to be first-generation boarders. Can boarding complement family life? Can boarding provide an effective substitute when family life is dysfunctional? Discussion continues over this aspect of the *Children Act*'s philosophy.

With regard to the three foci of the *Children Act* (1989), child welfare is clearly the key concern of all settings but, as discussed in the context of the external environment, parental relationships, and therefore the opportunities for parental responsibility, vary considerably. Decision making involving young people is certainly best developed in the boarding schools and some special schools in which the more senior pupils may be given significant responsibility.

For some observers the position of prefect, or its equivalent, appears to open the door even wider to potential bullying or possibly abuse. However, the responsibilities entailed can represent progress in social development and as such are recognised in the National Minimum Standards for Boarding Schools (DoH, 2002e).

Child welfare

One focus of the *Children Act* (1989) is the directive that the welfare of the young person is paramount (Iwaniec and Hill, 1999) and takes precedence over all other considerations including loyalty to colleagues, and is the main consideration when courts are making decisions. Furthermore, a person who has care of a young person, but not parental responsibility, should do what is reasonable in all circumstances for the purpose of promoting or safeguarding the young person's welfare. Related to child protection, the Act covers a broad swathe of welfare topics including:

- health and safety regulations;
- actions to be taken in an emergency;
- confidentiality and data protection;
- accommodation and space requirements;
- hygiene;
- the care for sick young people;
- dietary considerations;
- security matters;
- religious observance;
- access to parents.

These are discussed elsewhere but confidentiality impinges directly upon the law and raises a number of concerns, since staff have a professional responsibility to share relevant information about child protection and other key welfare issues with other professionals. Should a young person ask for a confidential talk, the response must be that no guarantee of confidentiality may be given in that the disclosure may indicate other dangers or risks. In *Protecting Children* (DoH, 1988) it is clearly stated: 'the keeping of confidence in some cases can amount to maintaining the secret of abuse.' Therefore, staff should share information about young people and families on only a 'need to know' basis with appropriate professionals. However, apart from the pastoral and child protection aspects, confidentiality also has a medical and data protection connotation. In essence, the manager or responsible member of the residential staff has the authority to make medical disclosures if, without them, the young person is disadvantaged. However, should there be any doubt at all, it is best to seek the advice of an appropriate doctor.

A particularly difficult situation arises when the young person of sufficient age or competence does not wish medical information to be passed to those with parental responsibility. If, in the considered opinion of the manager, serious harm to the young person or to others may result from non-disclosure, the right of confidentiality can be set aside. In general terms, a young person over the age of 16 is, under appropriate circumstances, entitled to confidentiality of information. With the Gillick competencies (Allen, 1992), a young person under the age of 16, but judged to be of sufficient maturity and understanding, may also be so entitled.

Confidentiality is a complex subject and the role of residential staff is significantly different from that of medical doctors or priests. The sole judgement should be for the welfare of the young person involved and, as an act of self-preservation, the staff member should keep detailed records of all the circumstances. This raises the question of the *Data Protection Act* (1998) which sets out the conditions for the handling of data relating to individuals. Unless it is judged in some way harmful, young people of sufficient age or competence and those with parental responsibility can gain access to medical records. This right accords with the *Data Protection Acts* (1984 and 1988) and *Access to Health Records Act* (1990). Closely related is the question of consent for which the age of 16 and Gillick competencies also apply (Franklin, 2002).

Parental responsibility

A second overriding concern of the Act is for partnership with those who have parental responsibility (Davies, 1997). Therefore, for staff in residential and boarding education and care there is a need to bear constantly in mind the role and authority of parents and of their own limitations in acting *in loco parentis*.

When the *Children Act* (1989) came into force on 14 October 1991 the concept of parental responsibility came into being, subsuming the parental rights and duties of the *Children Act* (1975), and thereby altering the legal status of all parents. Parental responsibility may be shared but cannot be lost until the young person reaches the age of majority, is adopted or is freed for adoption (Allen, 1992). In Section 3 of the Act parental responsibility is defined as: 'all the rights, duties, powers, responsibilities and authority which by law a parent of a child has in relation to the child and his property.'

The rights of the child and the duties of the parent may change over time, particularly with regard to the competence of the young person to give consent. Parents, on the birth of their child, have parental responsibility unless they were unmarried at the time of or after conception in which case the mother alone has parental responsibility. The father can acquire responsibility through a court order or agreement (DoH, 1989b). Later in Section 2, the Act states: 'a person who has parental responsibility for a child may not surrender or transfer any part of that responsibility to another.' As a result, residential staff can have delegated parental responsibility, an authority delegated by the parents via the head or senior manager (Section 2 the *Children Act* (1989)).

The person who has parental responsibility can arrange for some or all of that responsibility to be met by one or more persons on his behalf. Such guardians may be appointed by parents or possibly by the establishment or an outside agency. If the establishment is involved, the appointment should be treated in a similar way to that for staff with a focus upon the CRB disclosure procedure.

The appointment of a guardian *ad litem* (DoH, 1991d) is a more specialised procedure, mandatory in 'specified proceedings' unless the court is satisfied that an appointment is not necessary in order to safeguard the child's interests (Allen, 1992). For all to whom such responsibility has been delegated there is a duty to safeguard and promote the welfare of each young person accommodated. Therefore, the situation can be complex and, in any residential setting, it is vital to check on the exact legal responsibility of those at various levels of management and to know who has delegated parental responsibility for a particular child. It is obviously important to keep records of all decisions made in the interests of the young person and to be able to defend them on the grounds that they were reasonable. There is a detailed discussion on this subject in Allen (1992) and Mitchels and Prince (1992).

In any setting, many young people have parents who are divorced so that parental responsibility is split. As a result, there may be difficulties with regard to agreement on access and staff must be aware of who has access. In cases in which there has been delegation, a careful record must be kept of what has been delegated. The care delegated may not, for example, include certain activities, external visits or medical treatment. Furthermore, parental delegation can be changed and records must therefore be current.

In addition to statutory power, the manager or residential staff member is *in loco parentis* under common law and, in most cases, has the consent of the parent or young person or both. If there are any doubts, signed permission needs to be obtained from the parents so that the manager can make decisions in the best interests of the young person and not under the threat of subsequent legal action. For parents abroad and children who are not competent to give their own consent, it is advisable to keep an in-date, signed general permission to be used in emergencies.

There are further complications in that the Act sets out new ways of sharing responsibility between separated parents with people outside the immediate family and with the Local Authority. It is vital that residential staff know of the arrangements which obtain and also of any specific orders. If there are any doubts about the court orders or indeed any of the other legal points, it is wise to take expert advice before proceeding.

The overall emphasis must be on partnership with families by:

- consulting and notifying parents about decisions affecting the child;
- promoting contact between the child and his parents and family where it is reasonably practicable and consistent with the child's welfare;
- seeking to work with the parents to achieve a safe and stable environment for the child to return to (where this is judged feasible) or by finding a satisfactory alternative placement for the child.

(DoH, 1991a).

Decision making

The third point emphasised in the Act is decision making involving young people. Young people should be involved, as far as possible, in making the important decisions about their own lives. If they are aged 16 and over, they have the right to give or withhold consent and, below the age of 16, the right may be granted as a result of Gillick competence. However, if consent is refused in a medical situation, the final decision rests with the doctor.

These issues are all at the more extreme end of decision making and are likely to occur relatively rarely. The aim of the *Children Act* (1989) is to encourage consultation with young people and the establishment of a participative environment for the setting. Young people should be encouraged to take increasing responsibility for their own appearance and behaviour. Transitions from a dependent status towards independence, discussed in Chapter 5, are identified by behaviours related to personal and social development. For the transfer of real responsibility to young people to be a realistic possibility, the length of stay in residence would need to be relatively long. In boarding schools, the more senior and mature young people tend to be given enhanced rights and responsibilities. However, in other settings, even if such a procedure may not rival that in boarding schools, more limited responsibilities may be delegated during the course of living and learning. This is evident in many of the token systems which reward good behaviour and trust. Indeed, trust must be one of the most important relationships between staff and young people in that it is only with a degree of trust that any residential establishment can run smoothly and beneficially for all the young people.

The reverse face of rewards is of course sanctions, a subject which raises considerable controversy. Initially, the point is whether good behaviour is rewarded and bad behaviour is punished or whether, in the interest of emphasising only the positive, bad behaviour is ignored. The former might seem to represent a 'fairer' situation. Enhancement of the good must be applauded but what is the effect of punishment? Does punishing bad behaviour improve the situation for the individual? What are the effects upon the remainder of the young people? It would be generally agreed that punishment should not represent retribution. Sanctions may also be viewed as part of rehabilitation. For example, they may take the form of reparation to the victim or at least some form of recompense. Restorative justice as an antidote to recidivism is being tried in a number of settings. It is possible to develop these arguments in various ways but it would be reasonable to conclude that the aim must be longer term benefit for the child or young person. Punishment, in whatever form, is most justifiably awarded in the context of later rehabilitation. Punishment to ensure fairness is a beguiling argument but since all the young people will be different, what exactly constitutes fairness? Fairness must be a question of debate. Should the punishment fit the crime or the person who committed the crime?

Strict guidelines on permissible forms of control have been issued (DoH, 1993). These controls are based upon permitted disciplinary measures and prohibited measures set out in the *Children Act* (1989) (DoH, 1991a). The prohibited measures are: corporal punishment, deprivation of food and drink, restriction or refusal of visits/communications, requiring a young person to wear distinctive or inappropriate clothing, the use or the withholding of medication or medical or dental treatment, the use of accommodation to physically restrict the liberty of any child, intentional deprivation of sleep, imposition of fines, and intimate physical searches. In the National Minimum Standards for Boarding Schools, the fact that corporal punishment is no longer permissible is set out in Standard 4:

> No unacceptable, excessive or idiosyncratic punishments are used by boarders or staff, including any punishment intended to cause pain, anxiety or humiliation, corporal punishment.

It would appear that with regard to permissible controls, there is agreement across the field of residential and boarding education and care as to what is not permitted. It may be taken that permitted measures (DoH, 1991a) enjoy an equal degree of agreement. They may be summarised as follows:

- approval and rewards;
- verbal reprimand;
- reparation and compensation of no more than two-thirds of the young person's pocket-money;
- curtailment of leisure extras;
- additional household chores;
- increased supervision.

Complaints procedure

Whatever the setting, the complaints procedure provides a clear indication that welfare is paramount and there is the potential for the young people to exercise a degree of control over what happens to them. The procedure empowers the young people, and thereby alters the balance between them and those directly responsible for their care. In *Guidance and Regulations. Volume 5: Independent Schools* (DoH, 1991b), the complaints procedure is described as follows:

> It is important that there should be clear and accessible avenues for children to alert an appropriate adult to situations which are causing them distress.

The exact procedure will vary according to sector but it needs to cover not only child protection but also welfare rights and social justice rights. The complaints procedure therefore complements the main thrust of the *Children Act* (1989) by providing a practical outlet for the young people. A disclosure of abuse may be seen as a specialised form of complaint.

A framework for the procedure is provided in *Guidance Regulations. Volume 4: Residential Care* (DoH, 1991a). Any definite complaint, whether formal or informal, should be recorded and it is good practice to present the response, even to an informal complaint, in writing. If the complaint passes beyond the informal stage a person who is independent of the establishment should always be involved as an objective witness in the considerations. The procedure is broadly based in that, apart from the young person or those with parental responsibility, anybody judged to have sufficient interest in the young person's welfare can make a complaint on that young person's behalf. Thus the procedure may spill over into the field of advocacy.

The full procedure should be well known to members of the residential staff and to all the young people. It is appropriate to appoint a senior member of staff as the designated person for such complaints. That person needs to keep a record of complaints and to ensure that the entire procedure is given a high level of confidentiality.

While the complaints procedure must be set out clearly in the documentation of the establishment, it will, by its nature, merge into the child protection and anti-bullying procedures. At the informal stage, it is likely to overlap with daily mechanisms for considering minor issues. The young people should be encouraged to express their feelings and the staff should help explore the concerns to achieve some form of agreed understanding. If at all possible, a satisfactory outcome should be found through mediation.

For the young people, the procedure is part of the pastoral care system but is distinguished by the fact that a complaint can be clearly defined. A complaint is specific and focused and of sufficient relevance to the young person to have been preceded by a certain amount of thought. During the procedure, there is obvious scope for outside support of the young person from counsellors, advocates or independent visitors. As described in *Introduction to the Children Act* (DoH, 1989b), independent visitors, or others acting in a similar role, should achieve a balance in that they should not be complete strangers to the young people but should be divorced as far as possible from the hierarchy of the establishment. They need to be familiar to the young people if approaches are ever to be made for their services but they must be covered by a CRB clearance and be known by the staff to explain their presence in the establishment. This balance is managed in a variety of ways in the different settings. An approach common to secure units, children's homes and boarding schools is to have a formal introduction at the start of a young person's period of residence. The young person and the independent visitor can then be left to make their own arrangements for communication and meetings. Thereafter, the visitor arrives at the request of the young person and has only the minimum necessary contact with residential staff.

That the complaints procedure raises a variety of issues is apparent from the different ways it is tackled in the various establishments. In some it tends to be seen as a specific procedure whereas in others it is envisaged more broadly as giving the young people a voice in all aspects of their welfare. Depending upon which approach is taken, so the number of complaints recorded may be interpreted in different ways. If there are very few complaints, it may mean that the establishment runs very well and the young people are more or less completely happy, or it may indicate that the regime is so authoritarian that only a few dare to complain. Many complaints would seem to show that there are many problems but they also indicate an open society in which the young people are encouraged to think and act for themselves. In any environment with young people and staff living and learning together there are bound to be general grumbles and complaints, and the key factor must be the nature of the complaint.

Care Standards Act (2000)

Almost the entire field of residential and boarding education and care became the subject of National Minimum Standards in April 2002. Service Standards were published for the following: children's homes, residential special schools, boarding schools, FE colleges (accommodation of students under age 18 by FE colleges) and care homes for younger adults. There are also Standards for custodial care, produced by the Custodial Care National Training Organisation (2002) and for Child and Adolescent Psychiatric In-Patient Services produced by the Quality Network for In-Patient CAMHS (Child and Adolescent Mental Health Services) (2001). In addition, the Charterhouse Group published, as an adjunct to those for children's homes, Standards for therapeutic community child care, health and education. Standards are intended to provide nationally defined minimum standards for the provision of welfare in a particular setting so that:

- the same National Minimum Standards should apply to all young people in a particular sector of residence;
- welfare should be of good quality;
- the individual characteristics of the particular establishment, expressed through the mission statement or other document, should not be inhibited;
- Standards should be sufficiently specific to allow consistency in interpretation;
- Standards should be derived from other appropriate standards or relevant government guidance.

Few would deny the need for such Standards which form a basis for the inspection of residential education and care. However, the point about the characteristics of the individual establishment and its philosophy must always be borne in mind. For settings concerned chiefly with education, health or custodial care, Social Service procedures may have been largely unknown. However, since the implementation of the *Children Act* (1989) and particularly the accent upon child protection, good working relationships have normally been established. In general, children's homes, the residential settings with which Social Services are most familiar, are relatively small. Therefore, the size factor of many of the other establishments alone means that Social Service Inspectors are at least as apprehensive about carrying out the inspection as are the residential staff of being at the receiving end. It is hoped that the best practice developed jointly between the staff in the settings and the inspection teams will be continued by the new regional inspection teams established as a result of the implementation of the *Care Standards Act* in April 2002.

All the sets of Standards cover much the same ground although distinctive sources can be discerned. For example, the boarding schools and FE college Standards are derived from the same basic set which is different from that used for the generation of the residential special school and children's home Standards. The former are broadly based with an accent upon education and the latter are very much concerned with care. The Standards for young people in care homes derive from a third source in that they have been developed alongside care Standards for adult care homes. These five sets of Standards however have a great deal in common and it would seem reasonable to hope that in the future one general set of Standards combining the best of each might suffice, with a few extra specialised Standards for each setting. It must be remembered that young people with very similar backgrounds may be found in each of these five types of setting. Custodial Care Standards include a number of elements not required in any of the others and the psychiatric care Standards are concerned predominantly with health matters. However, they all have an underlying theme of people, premises and policies. Therefore, they are in many ways comparable and they do indicate scope for the transfer of good practice from one sector to another.

Each National Minimum Standard comprises three elements:

1   The Standard.
2   The outcome.
3   Criteria for judging the Standard.

The inclusion of an outcome is apparently to match general DoH practice despite the fact that in many cases 'outcome' means 'desired outcome'. For example, the realistic outcome with regard to anti-bullying procedures should be that satisfactory procedures and policies are in place and cannot be that there is no bullying, a situation which can never be guaranteed. However, while the outcome has raised discussion, the criteria cause definite problems.

There are four main sources of evidence open to inspectors: observation, interviews, discussion, and documentation. The evaluation should be positive while attempting to identify shortcomings, and criteria should allow comparisons to be made with comparable settings. Rather than listing specific criteria for each standard, it might have been preferable to allow the inspectors in the field to select the appropriate method. As matters stand, many of the criteria are impossible to evaluate. For example, a criterion which commences: 'Staff know that ...' can be assessed in a small establishment but in a boarding school or FE college, other than through a detailed survey, it would be extremely difficult to ascertain whether all the staff do know and what in fact 'knowing' actually means.

There are obvious measurables such as the presence or absence of a policy and the space around each bed but there are so many criteria, particularly in the Standards for boarding schools and FE colleges in which definition of what is required poses problems. Words such as 'suitable', 'appropriate', 'effective' and 'fair' occur commonly and can be assessed only subjectively. A further interesting issue concerns assessment criteria which involve the young people. If judgement is to be by the young people, laudable as such a procedure may seem, there are major difficulties in any moderately large-scale establishment. It is interesting that most criteria to be judged by the young people occur in the boarding school Standards, significantly fewer in the FE college Standards and effectively none at all in the remainder. To obtain the views of the young people in a children's home would not normally be too difficult whereas to carry out the same procedure in a boarding school with several hundred young people would require a detailed and well-planned survey. If anonymous letters are used or reliance is placed upon casual disclosure during the inspection, the survey is hardly likely to be unbiased.

The number and focus of the Standards varies considerably according to the sector. For boarding schools there are fifty-two Standards of which sixteen are on general welfare and thirteen on premises. For FE colleges there are forty-seven Standards with a similar focus. For children's homes there are thirty-six Standards, the majority about care and only four about environment (premises). For residential special schools there are thirty-three Standards, of which twelve are directly on planning for and quality of care and only four on premises. For care homes for younger adults, the majority of Standards are concerned with the choice of home, individual needs and choices and lifestyle. Of particular interest in this set is Standard 9 on risk taking: 'Staff enable service users to take responsibility for risks, ensuring they have good information on which to base decisions', and Standard 11 on personal development: 'Staff enable service users to have opportunities to maintain and develop social, emotional, communication and independent living skills.'

On the subject of relationships between staff and young people, the core of the living and learning environment, there is only one Standard for boarding schools and FE colleges. This may be used to illustrate further the intrinsic differences between the sets of Standards. For boarding schools, the outcome is: 'There are sound relationships between staff and boarders.' The criteria include:

1   There are sound staff–boarder relationships.
2   The general view of boarders is that the staff look after them well and fairly, and the communication between staff and boarders is positive.

For FE colleges the same Standard is worded slightly differently. The outcome remains: 'sound relationships between staff and students' but the main criterion is: 'There are sound staff–student relationships including an understanding of respective roles, rights and responsibilities.' In sharp contrast, the children's home Standard for the same subject has the following outcome: 'Children enjoy sound relationships with the staff based on honesty and mutual respect.' The main criterion is: 'Relationships between staff and children are based on mutual respect and understanding and clear professional personal boundaries which are effective for both the individuals and the group.' It is strange that some Standards for boarding schools, with their strong accent on pastoral care and personal and social development, seem less appropriate for them than the Standards published for children's homes, residential special schools and care homes for young adults. Suffice it to say that the most compelling definitions of the human environment occur in the Standards for therapeutic community child care, health and education under the heading 'Defining characteristics of the therapeutic community concept':

• a shared commitment of the goal of learning from the experience of living and/or working together (living and learning situation);
• there is a living and learning culture where interdependence emerges through take-up of responsibilities rather than through the demand for rights.

Occupational Standards, concerned with the roles of staff at different levels within the establishment, have been produced for the custodial care sector and for managers in residential child care. They are set out in the same format as that used for the National Vocational Qualification (NVQ) documentation and comprise the following parts:

• the Standard, a simple statement of practice;
• the elements which make up the Standard;
• the performance criteria for each element;
• the range of competence required for each element;
• the knowledge, understanding and skills required for the Standard.

(TOPSS, 2003)

A narrow definition of residential child care has been adopted so that the management Standards are recognisable for children's homes but for few other settings. With relatively modest changes, they could be made generic for all residential and boarding education and care. This core set of Standards would then be supplemented by specialist occupational Standards appropriate to each setting.

Human Rights Act (1998)

The definitive update to the *Children Act* (1989) was provided by the *Human Rights Act* (1998) which brings into UK law much of the European *Convention on Human Rights*. This came into force on 2 October 2000 and it means that decisions must now be compatible with the European Convention, and this involves reinterpretation of existing legislation, rules and laws. A distinction is made, which is particularly useful in the residential environment, between the different types of rights which may be categorised as follows:

- absolute rights which include the right to life and the prohibition of degrading treatment;
- limited rights which cover liberty and security;
- qualified rights which involve freedom of thought, religion, expression and assembly.

The Act provides a strong underpinning for anti-discriminatory policy but it might also be invoked against rules or possibly sanctions used in the establishment. The range of rights set out in the Act is very wide and will undoubtedly impinge upon the relationship between staff and young people but, over time, it is expected that a reasonable balance will be achieved.

Equal opportunities

Like child protection, non-discrimination is a basic legal requirement everywhere. However, in the residential setting discrimination can become particularly pernicious in that, for the victim, there is no escape. Furthermore, since the activities and routines of daily living are largely public, there are numerous opportunities for discrimination which may merge into bullying or even abuse. In a day school, young people may be observed principally following the curriculum in class time and leisure pursuits in the breaks. In residence, virtually all aspects of living are transparent, from getting up in the morning to going to bed at night, and opportunities for genuine privacy are usually limited. Therefore, it seems appropriate that equal opportunities should, like child protection, be considered sufficiently important to be a separately identified framework component.

'Equal opportunities' is accepted as a positive generic term covering all forms of anti-discrimination. Various UK Acts have addressed elements of discrimination but the turning point occurred when the European Convention on Human Rights (1998) came into force. In Article 14, discrimination is specifically prohibited:

> the enjoyment of the rights and freedoms set forth in this Convention shall be secured without discrimination on any grounds such as sex, race, colour, language, religion, political or other opinion, national or social origin, association with a national minority, property, birth or status.

Protection against discrimination was thereby extended well beyond all the rights previously enjoyed. In what can sometimes be a highly charged environment such as that of residence, anti-discrimination demands an integrated approach to combat not only the categories of discrimination but also the modes of discrimination at all levels. It must always be remembered that the full force of discrimination can only be felt by the young person against whom it is directed. The effective elimination of discrimination must depend ultimately upon those who live in the human environment, both staff and young people, but it will be supported and even demanded from the external environment through the law and local authority professionals.

In any community situation there is likely to be an in-group and an out-group. The main difference in structure is that the in-group is likely to have a tightly bound core with some others more loosely attached while the out-group may comprise individuals and possibly small unattached groups. It appears endemic to group living that distinctions will be made which will cause some young people to bond together and others to be mainly outside the grouping. This may not represent positive discrimination but may be inadvertent in that the young person involved has little in common with those in the group.

Bonding factors or cultural currency ranges from sporting ability and physical attributes to personal variables such as appearance and sense of humour. It is particularly instructive for staff to know which variables do bestow cultural currency in their particular environment. On the personality spectrum, some young people will be located towards the introversion end and others towards the extraversion side and this is likely to be another factor affecting grouping. Some who are not in groups may indeed enjoy their isolation and remain totally unmoved by it. For others, it will remain a constant reminder that they are not popular and could be seen as a form of institutional bullying. However, groups change, depending upon the location and the activity, and it may be possible for staff to organise proceedings so that each of the young people is included in at least one group.

This discussion spills over into the question of group work and group dynamics. What can be done to integrate isolates? In that they lack the immediate support of their contemporaries, isolates run the risk of entering a descending spiral of increasing isolation and problems (Callow, 1994). Peer group learning and support is seen as increasingly crucial in residential living in all settings. The isolate may not be reminded of a particular duty or event and will not be sustained by the group when there are institutional or personal problems. The issue also involves consideration of group size, group values and the social development of the young people. Ultimately, it can impinge upon the ethos of the human environment and therefore the establishment, and may, of course, result in discrimination, bullying or even abuse, all of which raises the important question of staff intervention, discussed in Chapter 2. This needs to be enacted in a subtle way if any benefits are not to be undone once the member of staff has left the scene. To the group, the benefits of integration must be seen to outweigh, for whatever reason, the difficulties.

Discrimination

The main sources of possible discrimination with regard to the young people are:

- culture;
- gender;
- sexual orientation;
- ethnicity;
- language;
- disability;
- religion.

(Thompson, 1997)

In addition, there are the categories identified in the definition of discrimination given in the *Human Rights Act* (1998). There are also the more subtle forms of discrimination in the hazy area between discrimination and bullying or abuse. Discrimination may vary in intensity from the unintentional, inadvertent misuse of a word or possibly a discriminatory remark, to a display of positive prejudice. The former can be addressed in the personal, social and health education (PSHE) programme in school and by residential staff with a personal prompt, but the latter must be the subject of well-established policies and procedures within the establishment. Apart from a published policy which is familiar to all staff and young people, every effort needs to be made to develop a non-discriminatory atmosphere within the establishment so that any display of prejudice is seen to be out of keeping. As with abuse and bullying, support should be available for both the victim and the perpetrator. Furthermore, it is important that any sanction should not further alienate the perpetrator and the victim, but should, if possible, provide some benefit for the community. As with all complaints and serious problems, it is important to retain full documentation.

Bearing in mind their similarities, it is not surprising that discrimination, bullying and, to a certain extent, abuse have much in common in their modes of operation. Discrimination can be physical through assault or removal of property. More commonly it is likely to be verbal and the question then arises as to the intention. One instance might be considered discrimination whereas for it to constitute bullying there would normally need to be repetition. The offending words might be written perhaps in a note or as graffiti. Non-verbal discrimination comprises attitudes, actions and gestures including exclusion. These may also constitute bullying or emotional abuse. Indeed, the term 'emotional' covers an array of discrimination, bullying and abuse in that the apparent intention is to attack the inner being of the victim. Apart from sexual abuse, this may be the most lingering of all attacks upon an individual. In addition, it is the most difficult for staff to discern and address. Emotional pressure is likely to be exerted by one young person on another away from the view of any staff and it must be realised that staff intervention may only exacerbate the situation.

The effects of discrimination are that the individual is to an extent disempowered and may suffer a decline in self-esteem (Thompson, 1997). The result of this can be further discrimination, more prejudice, increasing isolation and depression, or even contemplated or actual suicide. Discrimination is extremely serious and can be fully appreciated only by those against whom it has been perpetrated. Furthermore, in a group situation, there is always the danger that those on the edge will take part in the hope of deflecting attention from themselves. In the longer term, bitterness and alienation may exercise a considerable influence on later life. It is also clear that in whatever form it occurs, discrimination is likely to damage the ethos and effectiveness of the establishment.

In conducting risk assessments, residential staff must avoid a deterministic attitude in that discrimination may not be easily forecast and their behaviour may result in self-fulfilling actions among the young people. Some of the categories of discrimination are malleable and even changeable whereas others are fixed. Culture can change through absorption or integration into a different culture. Language problems can be overcome by study and from increasing familiarity with the common language. Some disabilities may be cured or at least the effects upon the individual concerned may be minimised. Religion clearly can be changed but, with politics, constitutes perhaps the most potentially volatile issue in any group. However, any changes made should clearly be according to the wishes of the individual and not through duress. It is important that differences are discussed and, however deeply felt the aversions may be, no individual should be the target of discrimination.

Diversity

The need for equality is set out in the law and it is important that not only the policies and procedures but particularly staff attitudes and actions should all indicate that equality is the accepted norm in the establishment. This raises the interesting discussion of the relationship between equality and diversity. All the young people should enjoy equality but diversity can be celebrated. If differences between individuals are given prominence and used as part of the living and learning environment, then in a sense those individuals may be viewed as targets for potential discrimination. In residential and boarding education and care there is likely to be a random mix of potentially discriminating characteristics in the population, particularly among the young people but increasingly among the staff. It is reasonable to assume therefore that such diversity should be treated in a positive way. The differing interests, knowledge and skills of each group provide opportunities for all the young people to capitalise. Acquaintance with different cultures represents preparation for living in a multicultural world (Millam, 1996). Gender differences bring a range of benefits not only academically but also in cultural pursuits. Differences in sexuality may be understood in a non-predatory environment. New languages introduce new literature and culture. The problems of the disabled can act as a catalyst for support from the other young people. As important, they can learn when support is not required. Variations among the young people may be used for the benefit of all, even if this involves some positive discrimination. The increased awareness which can result over time should bring positive collective action so that discrimination is eliminated.

However, where stereotyping and discrimination persist, more positive action may be required. One interesting and apparently successful approach is through philosophy and the development of logical thinking. It is assumed that the actions of the young people, whether in discrimination, bullying or abuse, are for them, at the time of perpetration, rational. Logical thinking should indicate that, with introspection, there could be different rationalities involved and an outcome which is not inimical to either party may be selected. If there is a deeply ingrained mindset, this method provides a possibility for change.

Philosophy/aims/ethos

The fourth framework component is the only control generated internally. In fact, outside agencies or governing bodies will provide guidance for the philosophy but ideally it needs to be agreed by the staff and accepted by the young people. The philosophy is required by the Standards in the form of a statement of principles, and elsewhere it is set out in prospectuses and staff handbooks and as the mission statement. It incorporates the fundamental values, ideas and concepts which govern the life of the community. These may be linked in a long tradition going back perhaps to the Rule of St Benedict or they may be produced by the latest principal, head or manager as managerial current philosophy. Since they provide guidelines and justify purpose, they need to have a visionary element, taking in more than a short-term view, but also to be suggestive of application. The vision may never become reality but the establishment should benefit from the journey towards its realisation.

The philosophy is translated into aims and objectives. The aims indicate the direction the establishment wishes to take and its priorities. Examples would be: to prepare the young people for life and to help all the young people to realise their potential. These show clearly what the establishment is trying to do but the realisation of such aims can never be truly evaluated since the terminology renders them impossible to assess. Therefore, it can never be said that the aims have been fully achieved. At what stage can a young person be said to be prepared for life? Since each life will be unique and the vagaries of life cannot be forecast, such an aim represents a good intention. Similarly, potential is impossible to anticipate with any degree of accuracy. The question might also be asked: At what stage of life might it have been achieved?

The objectives constitute, in a sense, the milestones towards the aims. What type of behaviour indicates progress towards an aim? Objectives are susceptible to some form of measurement and therefore achievement can be discerned. A basic example might be that each young person can use a personal computer to a certain standard. This might be considered a milestone towards the enhancement of self-esteem and personal organisation leading to independence. This will obviously help on the route of preparation for life. The aims and their contributory objectives are then set out in policies, procedures and modes of operation. The priority accorded each will vary depending on the perceived function of the setting. This may be any or several of the following: shelter, social necessity, hostel, treatment, educative or training. It will also be the philosophical trend which is likely to differ according to whether the establishment is traditional or progressive.

The achievement of the objectives represents progress towards the aims which signpost the fulfilment of the philosophy. The result may be described as the ethos of the establishment. The ethos includes the physical environment but is seen chiefly through the operation of the human environment.

Philosophy

As a framework component, philosophy is far less specific than the aspects of the law since it can embrace everything about residential living. In its enactment, it demonstrates the values of the setting. From work in a variety of residential establishments, a basic list of values has evolved, normally including the following: choice, privacy, respect, independence, rights and fulfilment (DoH, 1989a). Some combination of these is likely to be found in mission statements. For example, they look towards the young people achieving a satisfying and worthwhile independence in life. This is likely to be realised in an environment where the young people have the opportunity to develop self-esteem, to make their own decisions and to enjoy a wide range of social relationships. They also have a reasonable degree of privacy, are treated with respect and accorded their rights in a community where these values are generally upheld.

The philosophy is also likely to be related to the needs of young people which have been summarised in numerous documents. The basis for these inventories was, in most cases, the UN Convention on the Rights of the Child. The main principles of the Convention are that:

- there should be no discrimination;
- decisions about a child must always consider the child's best interests;
- children have the right to be consulted on all matters concerning them.

A comprehensive list of needs, set out in Chapter 4, was produced by Kahan (1994) as a result of the work of the Wagner Development Committee.

While the gist of these needs is likely to be included in a detailed philosophy, the distinguishing feature will probably be the visionary element which incorporates a long-term component. This might, for example, encourage the development of the young people towards a fulfilled, self-disciplined and virtuous life. This can be achieved through the pursuit of excellence in all endeavours, inspired by high ideals in a secure and supportive community which shares responsibility with those who have parental responsibility.

Aims

The philosophy provides the basis for the aims which, although they cannot be directly assessed, should provide a complete and accurate guide to the direction that the establishment is taking. The Strategic National Objectives for Children and Young People (2003), in that they cannot be measured, are aims or direction indicators:

- health and emotional well-being: being healthy and feeling good;
- staying staff: being safe, feeling safe and reducing risks;
- fulfilment: getting the most out of life as a child and as a adult;
- social engagement: making a contribution and being a positive citizen;
- material well-being: having sufficient income to take advantage of opportunities.

These indicators are intended to provide the basis for the education, care and welfare of all young people. It is clear that they go beyond adolescence and it might be said that they have a fairly obvious political underpinning. The first three summarise what might be set out in more detail as the aims of residential and boarding education and care. Even so, there may well be criticism in that fulfilment also comes from putting the most into life. Economic well-being and positive citizenship would be subsumed, it might be thought, under fulfilment and preparation for life. Whether a young person becomes a positive citizen with sufficient income may depend upon a number of things well beyond an individual's control.

Each setting will have its own aims, ideally agreed as a result of a collaborative effort between staff and with some involvement from the young people. In this context, while it is reasonable to include the young people in such decision making, it must be remembered that they are temporary residents whereas many members of staff will represent something more stable. Furthermore, there is an essential difference in that the staff are there to teach and the young people to learn, although in the true spirit of a living and learning community there is some mutual exchange. The aims will vary even within a type of setting which is centrally controlled such as YOIs. If the aims, as stated, do not appear to show very much variation, there will be differences in interpretation and emphasis. The aims must also take into account the probable destination of the young people, whether it is into life, back to mainstream day schooling or possibly into a life of incarceration. The time factor is also critical in that aims must necessarily be restricted if the expected length of residence is short. In two months it is unrealistic to promulgate a series of lifetime aims. However, over several years in residence much can be achieved and preparations for life can be reasonably addressed.

Ethos

Progress through the achievement of objectives towards the aims of the establishment produce the ethos, atmosphere or climate. To those with experience of the different sectors of residential and boarding education and care, the ethos is tangible although elusive to describe. Furthermore, it can be fully identified only as a result of a period of residence in the establishment. It is influenced initially by the surroundings and the built environment. The various areas within the establishment – personal, shared, domestic, recreational and administrative – all add to the overall feeling. The effect upon the observer is produced by a combination of many variables discussed in the context of the physical environment; for example, the state of the fabric, the décor, decorations and the attitude towards the built environment of the young people. However, the overriding aspects which govern the ethos are concerned with the human environment. How are the values which contribute to the philosophy apparent in the way the community operates? The relationships between the young people and between them and the staff also provide strong indicators which affect the climate of the setting. The level of formality, the respect shown and the courtesies exchanged all indicate something of the environment. If there is no clear ethos indicating a caring and supportive human environment, the aims and possibly the philosophy require re-examination.

It is possible to evaluate the objectives directly since these represent measurable units. The assessment of aims can therefore be made within a certain probability in the short term but only more debatably in the long term. The only valid approach for the latter would be through a longitudinal study such as the 1958 British Cohort Study (Shepherd, 1997). Inspections result in the evaluation of objectives through observation, interviews, discussions and documentation. For each setting, there are likely to be general assessments of success such as examination results, improved behaviour, non-recidivism, military or other skills, and cured or improved medical conditions. Furthermore, it has been demonstrated that personal and social development characteristics can be reliably and validly assessed using the technique discussed in Chapter 5. However, it must be remembered that, in the words of Sir William Utting: 'the factors determining human behaviour are so many and variable, and so difficult to measure, that "answers" are rarely certain and at best probable' (Soisson, 1992). Sir William goes on to say that this need not cause embarrassment since for social workers insights from 'soft' observations can be just as useful as the findings of 'hard' research.

Chapter 4

Developmental components

The interplay of the environmental components, governed by the framework components, provides a summary of living together and learning together at any one instance. Over time, change occurs, particularly in the young people. Such change results partly from internal factors concerned with maturation and partly through the environment. Depending upon the setting and related variables such as length and continuity of stay, the residential and boarding education and care environment can claim more or less responsibility for changes in the young people. If residence is long and virtually continuous, the establishment must have prime responsibility. If the stay is short or intermittent, change may be attributed more to those who have parental responsibility.

Change in a young person is characterised as development and is apparent in many aspects of life and behaviour: personal, social, spiritual, sexual, moral, emotional, educational and physical. For the model, these comprise the developmental components. However, through research and discussion, the inventory has been reduced to five components. Depending upon fullness of definition, there remains some overlap but these five have proved sufficiently discrete and robust for staff training.

The fundamental purpose of residential education is to address the needs of the young people who live in each setting. There are immediate needs and longer term needs, particularly concerning life after residence, and these should be covered by the aims and objectives and addressed by the practices of the establishment. The key to residential education is the preparation of the young people for the next stage of life; for young people in the children's home or special school this may be a return to the family home and mainstream schooling. In a boarding school, some special schools and many of the other types of setting it may be further or higher education. In a forensic psychiatric setting it may be a lifetime of incarceration while in custodial care it may be integration into society or a further period in custody.

Perhaps the best-known statement on children's needs is that set out by Kellmer Pringle (1975). Apart from physical care, the inventory is:

- the need for love and security;
- the need for new experiences;
- the need for praise and recognition;
- the need for responsibility.

For residential settings, Maier (1987) identified the ingredients of the common core of caring, the key points of which were the following:

- bodily comfort;
- differentiating between individuals;
- predictability;
- dependability;
- training in personal behaviour;
- care for the care givers.

This list involves the needs of children with implications for the residential staff and offers key points for the ethos of the establishment.

Among the most complete inventories is that set out in Kahan (1994):

> Physical comfort, shelter, warmth and food; a stable environment to live in and to feel safe and secure; protection from abuse and ill-use; proper health care; education and the opportunity to fulfil their potential; personal privacy and space; association with, and the opportunity to make friends with children of their own age; to feel valued by other people, particularly those who are significant to them like parents or substitute parents; and clear boundaries, consistency in the care they receive and effective benevolent control.

These general needs are common to all young people and beyond these are the specific needs of particular groups which differ according to a number of variables, principally: family and environment, health, social factors and educational requirements.

In its guide, the DoH (2000a and 2000b) includes an assessment framework for the needs of children. The needs are classified into three broad categories:

1   Children's developmental needs.
2   Parenting capacity.
3   Family and environmental factors.

The third category does not impinge directly on the operation of residential and boarding education and care except through the interaction with the external environment. The young person's developmental needs are listed as: health, education, emotional and behavioural development, identity, family and social relationships, social presentation and self-care skills. Parenting capacity comprises: basic care, ensuring safety, emotional warmth, stimulation, guidance, and boundaries and stability. These identified needs vary considerably in character (Horwath, 2001).

On the basis of the Maslow (1943) hierarchy, health, basic care and ensuring safety are fundamental for survival. Once survival is assured, personal development, social development and then education follow. From the DoH (2000a and 2000b) list, health and education are major subjects whereas stimulation and stability are highly desirable benefits of family life without which many young people have to live. Basic care is essentially a staff input whereas identity may be related more closely to the outputs of the system since one purpose of residential living is to enhance self-esteem. While health and education involve obvious staff inputs, they are key outcomes.

In general, the young person's developmental needs, as listed, can be refashioned as aims for the young people in residential living. The factors of parenting capacity, set out in the DoH publications, can be similarly developed, but as staff aims. However, it is clear that staff are likely to have major inputs into many of the developmental needs and some inputs into all of them.

These issues illustrate the problem of attempting a universally accepted classification. The difficulty is compounded by the fact that certain needs are made implicit whereas others are subsumed. For example, in the assessment framework, moral development does not occur. It is obviously related to behaviour, relationships and social presentation but many will consider that it is something more. A further important issue is that the achievement of the related aims and objectives is, in some cases, clearly susceptible to some form of evaluation but in others less so. There are well-developed measures for health and education but not for identity or social presentation. With regard to parenting capacity, basic care can be assessed relatively easily whereas stimulation depends not only upon staff action but upon the personality of the young person involved. However, some form of evaluation is important if the effectiveness of the establishment is to be gauged.

In systems terms, residential and boarding education and care tends to be viewed as a black box, and the relationship between what goes on within the establishment and the outcomes has been resistant to research in depth. The Dartington Social Research Unit, after many years of research in various types of residential care for young people, has developed for children's homes evidence for the relationship of structure and culture to outcomes. The measures devised are essentially subjective but are based upon procedures for incidents. For example, many of the events of the daily round such as mealtimes and bedtimes will be conducted significantly differently in an authoritarian rather than a more democratic environment. Questions of structure and culture clearly overlap with the needs of young people in that they are assessed by outcomes for the young people, but are related more directly to the operation of the environmental components (Brown *et al.*, 1998).

The development of the young people's needs must indicate an alternative, if complementary, method of assessing an establishment. The issue is how, from the many differing classifications of children's needs, it is possible to produce a limited but comprehensive set of developmental components which allow at least a degree of measurement. The nineteen distinct settings in which young people live away from home in groups address health, social, educational and custodial issues. Each focuses upon care, health and education but whereas in all the settings the needs of the young people are paramount, in custodial establishments they are probably matched by other aims related to the law, punishment and the removal of individuals from society. With the increasing accent upon rehabilitation through the work of the YJB, this group of settings will become less distinctive. Already, the fact that inmates under the age of 18 have been brought under the aegis of the *Children Act* (1989), indicates welcome changes in approach. Their inclusion under the legislation highlights the fact that the UK government in ratifying the United Nations *Convention on the Rights of the Child* set out a number of reservations among which was the fact that the minimum ages for service in the armed forces are 16 years for young men and 17 years for young women. The Convention had required that priority be given to the recruitment of young people over the age of 18 years. As a result, the military training establishments are not included in the categories of residential education and care covered by the *Children Act* (1989).

Although they are clearly interrelated in many ways, care, health and education offer distinctive components of the needs of young people and are therefore key elements of development. However, although these three undoubtedly contribute significantly, they do not totally cover the emotional, spiritual, moral, personal and social aspects of development. Particularly in a residential setting where, by definition, family inputs are limited if not in some cases eliminated, consideration of personal and social development (PSD) is vital. The term 'PSD' is taken to subsume the emotional, spiritual, moral and related areas of development (Coleman and Hendry, 1999). Over the last few years in schools, a number of cross-disciplinary, in some cases pastoral, subjects have been introduced. Among these is PSHE to which citizenship is sometimes added (PSHCE). For residential and boarding education and care, it is felt that since health is the main determinant of residence for a reasonable proportion of the population living away from home in groups, it should be separated from PSD. Furthermore, it is clearly a major subject in its own right.

Evidence of development is measured most effectively using the behaviour, defined in the widest possible terms, of the young person. This statement is perhaps least obvious in the case of the educational component but, even in that field, true understanding is best demonstrated by application. The point is made to distinguish behaviour as a very general term which describes the totality of the reactions of an organism in its environment and the more common use of the word, most obviously seen in the distinction between good behaviour and bad behaviour. Behaviour, in this second sense, is clearly a major consideration in custodial care settings. However, since residential education is group living, such behaviour is also of significance in all settings. As a result, it seems appropriate to identify behaviour as the fifth developmental component. While related to the other three, behaviour is linked most closely to PSD in that bad, unacceptable or antisocial behaviour is frequently cited as an indicator of some lack in personal development. Conversely, effective work in PSD should be paralleled by a change in behaviour. However, since behaviour, in the good or bad sense, in no way summarises all PSD and may itself be a focus of attention in most residential settings, it is justified to consider it as a separate component.

These five components – education, health (and medical), care (and welfare), PSD and behaviour – are judged to provide a summary of development (Figure 4.1). Their identification as such has been tested in numerous meetings and in a variety of presentations. No additional component has been advanced and the main caveat remains that there is some overlap. This must be accepted as it is in so many aspects of scientific classification. The boundaries are essentially artificial but they facilitate discussion about good practice, proposals for training and opportunities for research which, without them, would be unnecessarily complex.

It is interesting to note in this context that in what remains a landmark study on the development of the young people by Rutter et al. (1971), education, health and behaviour were identified as foci.

The most obvious overlap is that all five components are associated in the totality of education. This may be evidenced by a healthy lifestyle, an independence in self-care, a realistic estimate of self-esteem and a reasonable level of social behaviour. If each is considered to be a black box (Chapter 1), this same point may be illustrated by the inputs and outputs (Figure 4.2). For education, the inputs include the National Curriculum and citizenship, and the outputs academic performance and certain elements of lifestyle. For health, there are many medical and health care inputs specific to the individual and the outputs include health and a healthy lifestyle. For care, primary care, personal care and security are among the inputs, and confidence and good self-presentation are examples of outputs. For behaviour, behaviour modification in some form may be among the inputs and improved behaviour among the outputs. Most of these outputs may be related to PSD for which examples of inputs are residential education itself, pastoral care and counselling, and outputs include an array of personal and social characteristics and qualities such as self-reliance, self-esteem, independence and the ability to form good relationships. Seen in this light, PSD pervades the other four components but is sufficiently important and distinct to provide a focus of its own. Furthermore, it is what many would consider to be the essence of residential education. PSD is also, in a sense, a higher order than the other components in that ultimately the quality of person who emerges from the system should be resilient and able to overcome deficiencies in the other components.

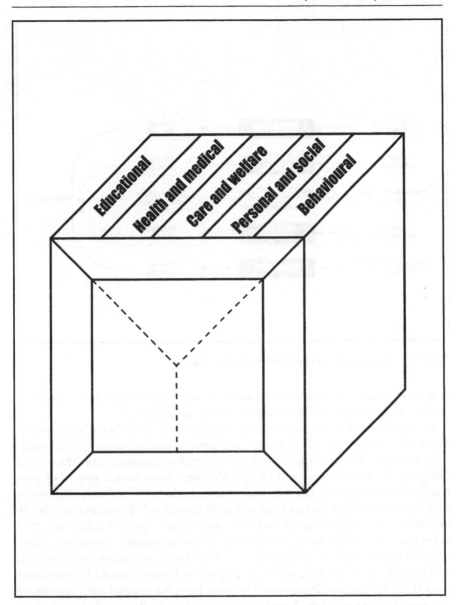

Figure 4.1   Developmental components

In the context of a systems approach, the division of the developmental aspect of residential and boarding education and care for young people into five components lightens the shade of the original black box in that, in assessing the progress of the young people, five developmental profiles and their

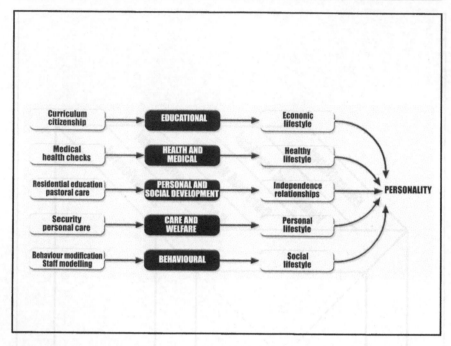

Figure 4.2   Developmental components as black boxes

interrelationship may be used. As each component is discussed, it is hoped that the five component boxes themselves can become grey boxes.

In considering the components, it is apparent that, while they provide a summary of development, they do not represent a homogeneous classification. Education, health and medical, and care and welfare summarise the three main components of any course and identify the three main interest groups of professionals involved in residential and boarding education and care. Behaviour may be seen as either very general or highly specialised. These four are clearly defined in their subject matter and the ways in which needs are addressed. PSD is far more difficult to define and therefore the measurement of progress is more difficult to assess. There are specialist residential settings which focus upon each of the other four components but not upon PSD, which should be integrated into all establishments. Professional support from the external environment, or in some cases as part of the human environment, is clearly provided for the four components but, for PSD except in the more extreme cases, it is not available. Teachers, medical staff, residential staff and various forms of therapist all operate in a clearly defined sector. Psychologists may be called in to address the more extreme problems associated with PSD. However, in general PSD is the one component for which there is almost total reliance on all the internal staff. All categories of staff associated with residential and boarding education and care can contribute.

For each of the components, progress is marked by stages of development separated by thresholds. For example, in education a threshold divides those young people who learn directly from the teacher and those who begin to take responsibility for their own learning. In health and medical there is the onset of puberty. In care and welfare, the threshold between dependence for some primary aspects of care and independence is relatively clear-cut. For behaviour, the development of introspection results in a threshold between those whose response is effectively a reflex action and those who respond in a more measured fashion. In the case of PSD the situation appears to be more complex. There are recognised thresholds separating an approach to life which is self-centred from that which is conforming and that which indicates independence. However, since these two thresholds may be seen in a variety of characteristics which make up PSD the thresholds for any two characteristics may not coincide. On a student profile or time-line for each of the five components, it would be more difficult to locate the thresholds for PSD than for any of the other components. Furthermore, if there is staff concern about progress, there is a portfolio of validated remedial measures available for all except PSD. For each component, a baseline position for each young person may be established using a variety of assessment procedures; these are least obvious in the case of PSD.

Not only are they closely interlinked, but the developmental components as a group relate closely to the other components identified in the model. Since development is measured by the monitoring and assessment of everyday life in the human environment, this is scarcely surprising (e.g. Fawcett, 1996). Some connections are less obvious. For example, the introduction of experts would involve the external environment. The subject matter of the components is covered, in some cases specifically and in others in more broad terms by the law. The end-product of development monitoring and assessment is seen in transitions. Indeed, transitions summarise development during the passage of the young person through the establishment.

Component 1: Educational

In the UK, all young people from the ages of 5 to 16 are required to attend school. For young people between the ages of 16 and 18, there is strong pressure through the DfES to undergo some form of training, if not FE, but no overt compulsion. For the school age group, to the age of 18 where applicable, in residential or boarding education and care there is a strong accent throughout on training and education. However, it is undeniable that the educational opportunities and the ingredients of the programmes will differ considerably among, for example, YOIs, military establishments, FE colleges and boarding schools. There are, of course, long-standing controversies as to the content of education as opposed to training or indeed vocational as opposed to academic education. The educational component is taken to cover all formal aspects of education and training which normally take place in designated teaching areas (Blyth and Milner, 1997).

This discussion raises the issue of responsibility for education. Where the facilities are an integral part of the establishment, responsibility is clear. In cases where the young people leave the setting to go to an external school, responsibility is shared. In school there is a different peer group and the pastoral or care system is likely to differ from that in the residential setting. For those with responsibility for the young people in the residential setting, special problems are therefore posed.

A further issue concerns residential and boarding education itself which should obviously contribute towards formal education but is in fact best seen in PSD. Residential and boarding education is seen as parallel and complementary to family life and parenting. Life skills are taught through the experience of everyday events. The parallel is very clear-cut in the case of settings which use external schooling. In those cases, the peer groups of the residents will include young people who return to their families at night. For settings in which the edu-cational facility is integral, the distinction between formal education and resi-dential education is less clear. For example, a teacher may also be involved as a member of the residential staff, a situation which is the norm in boarding schools. A virtual fusion of formal and residential education may occur at times during homework, whether in a residential setting or in a family. In assisting with homework, the residential staff or parents may well move from the aca-demic to the informal in their efforts to help. Nonetheless, by its nature, resi-dential education is considered more appropriately in the context of the PSD component and is particularly significant during the problems of adolescence (Varma, 1997).

What is the role of the member of the residential staff who is not also a teacher with regard to the education component? In any setting, whether or not the formal education is integral, the member of staff acts as a model. In the case of education, this entails having a good working knowledge of the education system in general and of where information may be obtained but, most impor-tant, never disparaging education. It is relatively easy to make a case for pro-grammes of specialised training such as motor mechanics, decorating or cooking, but the case for poetry or philosophy is more complicated. However, poetry through its inspirational qualities or philosophy through the develop-ment of logical thinking may have more long-lasting effects which are transfer-able than a specialist trade course (Thomson, 2002). Literacy and numeracy are fundamental as both academic and life skills. Their development by residential staff provides a good example of the way in which residential can support more formal classroom education.

Guidance and support, or pastoral care, for those young people attending an external school is a related function of the residential care work or pastoral care. In one respect, this is an extension of the same role in the residential set-ting. It may be necessary to offer support or even advocacy to the young person in the school or even the internal educational facility. In the case of settings which are separate from the school, it is vital to establish a close relationship with the appropriate members of the school staff so that the educational development of the young person may be enhanced and monitored in a way which supplements and complements everything that happens in school. The residential staff member therefore requires at least some knowledge of the curriculum, key stages, standard attainment tests (SATs), school Standards and particularly support services such as Connexions, work experience coordination, Behaviour Guidance, Educational Social Work, Learning Monitoring and Careers Consultancy. Most schools make some use of the services of their LEA and residential staff should be aware of these.

If the education component is primarily the responsibility of a facility within the establishment it is obviously easier to develop close liaison with the teaching staff. It is indeed through the teaching staff that services such as Connexions are likely to be delivered to the establishment. Part of the duty of support is to maintain careful records of the education of the young people through monitoring and assessment within the residential setting. This is clearly acting as would a reasonable parent in a family situation.

A further aspect of the role concerns safety and security. The more obvious areas include travel to school but also safety within school. In the residence there is far greater potential for control over contemporary hazards, and those leaving the residence on a daily basis must be prepared for issues concerned with smoking, drugs and alcohol to be encountered. To these may be added the negative facets of sexual relationships. Another contemporary consideration for which responsibility must be taken, predominantly within the residential setting, relates to computing and the internet (Purser, 1998). The restriction of access by the young people to undesirable information on the internet is now the subject of the official guidelines (e.g. Scottish Executive, 1999). The risks of the internet which could affect young people in residential and boarding education and care include personal safety and legal issues. The young people may be disturbed by the subject matter and there are serious risks involving child protection. Legal issues include harassment, defamation and libel, netiquette, credit care issues, copyright and intellectual property rights, and viruses and hacking. The guidelines state that establishments should have internet-use policies which take into account both supervised and unsupervised use. The policies should refer to child protection procedures, and guidelines for internet use should be displayed prominently. Internet access and arrangements should be included in staff training and should cover protection by filter and blocker. Internet and child safety issues should be kept under constant review. The subject raises a range of interesting questions. For example, is resistance to pornography best developed by a total ban on its viewing? In the absence of examples it is still possible to have a rational discussion on the subject. In a similar way, to engender an aversion to drugs, it is recognised that it is not necessary to have been a consumer.

Component 2: Health and medical

The aim of any residential setting must be to maintain and if possible improve the health and medical condition of each young person. Health refers to general well-being (Stock, 1991) and comprises:

- physical health covering the functioning of the body;
- mental health subsuming intellectual, psychological, emotional, spiritual and social health;
- societal health which refers to the environment in which the young person lives.

When for any reason health cannot be maintained, medical intervention is required. The residential staff are concerned with and should be reasonably knowledgeable about health (National Children's Bureau (NCB), 1999). They are neither medical practitioners nor professional health experts, but they should have sufficient basic knowledge and foresight to be able to make a reasoned judgement as to the seriousness of a medical problem and whether the requirement is for first aid, a nurse, a doctor or a hospital. Residential staff must also be able to talk to the young people about special issues or contemporary hazards, ranging from sex and AIDS to drugs. It tends to be assumed that such matters are addressed at home or in school although, in reality, the main source of information for many young people will be the peer group. Therefore, for those living away from home in groups, there is a real danger that their knowledge may be limited or factually incorrect. To ensure that this is not so is an important responsibility of residential staff (Cooke, 1994).

The establishment should have a health policy which would include:

- a description of the medical and health care provision, including services within the establishment and those located externally with which the setting is registered;
- detailed statements on the qualifications, operation and availability of all the professional medical staff who are either permanently within the establishment or attached to it;
- an inventory of available first aid and medication facilities including the security of the medicines and protocols for the administration of prescribed and non-prescribed medication;
- a statement setting out the freedom of choice for medical consultation and treatment available to the young people together with, for each young person, an inventory of past and current medical problems, allergies and treatments.

Young people have a right to health but this implies also a responsibility to attempt to maintain a healthy lifestyle. In residence, the lifestyle is to a greater or lesser degree controlled in that there is a daily programme of activities and a limited menu of food. The menu itself should presuppose healthy eating but the final choice is usually up to the young person. Adequate sleep, physical fitness and a range of interests to safeguard mental alertness are all prerequisites. The other factor of increasing importance is that there should be no indulgence in contemporary hazards such as smoking, alcohol abuse, solvent sniffing or drug taking. A dependence upon any of these habits is obviously inimical to a healthy lifestyle.

A healthy lifestyle is only likely to be practised, particularly after leaving the residence, if there is a culture of health awareness (Health and Safety Executive Books, 1993; Health and Safety Executive Commission, 1995). Like PSD and much of citizenship, this should pervade the entire curriculum although it will be a focus of PSHCE. It is also clearly a key part of residential education. Ideally, the family background of the young people should have laid the foundations for healthy living but this may not be the case. Therefore, for many there can be an advantage in residential education over family living. The other major learning source is of course the behaviour of the staff who should serve as models for a healthy and reasonable lifestyle. It is clear that the overall ambience of the establishment sets the tone for appropriate living and a holistic approach to health: physical, mental and societal. These various considerations illustrate how closely health is interlinked with education and care in the development of young people.

The medical development of the young people will be overseen by professionals, internal and external. The larger establishments such as many of the boarding schools will have a nursing staff and probably an infirmary. Smaller settings such as most children's homes need to use external provision although they should have a designated doctor. Residential establishments in the health care sector are likely to have, in addition, specialist support services depending upon the specific needs of the young people while nurses and teachers carry out the duties of residential staff.

There is a particularly important point with regard to staff. Those employed as nurses must be Registered General Nurses (RGNs) and should have experience suitable for the post. A staff member who is not registered in this way may still be employed as a matron or assistant and may administer prescribed or non-prescribed medication, in both cases according to previously agreed protocols.

However, since the overall welfare of the young people is a key responsibility of the residential staff, there needs to be close liaison with all the medical staff. The medical staff monitor change with regard to specific conditions. The residential staff note the progress or otherwise in the medical field so that they can relate it to all the other aspects of residential living. For example, a medical condition may be the root cause of a particular type of behaviour; it may inhibit educational progress, it may lead to greater dependency in care and welfare, and it may influence several aspects of PSD such as self-esteem and relationships.

Health, and in particular the pursuit of a healthy lifestyle, entails the medical staff, but its monitoring and assessment is part of the role of the residential staff (Mitchels and Prince, 1992). Among the more obvious thresholds is puberty, and this is likely to have an impact upon self-image and relationships in general. Sexual development brings a whole range of issues related to emotional and moral development. It is a task of the residential staff to support the young people so that they can develop the knowledge and skills to allow effective decision making at what is a time of very rapid change for them. It is also a period of dawning self-awareness, including the acceptance of mortality, and young people are likely to be highly sensitive and, at times, to exhibit atypical behaviour. If the various contemporary hazards complicate matters, the health and medical component can become the major strand in monitoring and assessment. In such a case it is likely to impact considerably on the other four developmental components.

Age-specific checks by staff include for various year groups: general health, height, weight, vision and blood pressure (NCB, 1999). Together with these and immunisation as appropriate, examples of health promotion include:

- Year 3: accident prevention, road safety, stranger danger, nutrition, care in sun;
- Year 7: relationships, exercise, smoking, dental care, puberty;
- Year 10: substance abuse, diet, exercise, sexual health, information on health services;
- Year 11: self-referral.

(NCB, 1999)

The role of staff as models for the young people is clearly of great significance if the ambience of the total establishment is to be effective. The direct influence will of course vary considerably according to the procedures of the establishment. For example, if residential staff take their meals with the young people, then each mealtime can be a learning experience involving all components of development (Central Council for Education and Training in Social Work (CCETSW), 1978). Verbal relationships between adults and between adults and young people will be demonstrated, reasonable table manners inculcated, food choice for healthy living illustrated, sensible behaviour demanded and the selection of conversation topic can be enriching.

It is presupposed in most residential establishments that indulgence in any of the contemporary hazards (Kahan, 1994) by members of staff should be at the very least highly controlled and in private. Certain indulgences are likely, of course, to lead to dismissal. At the lowest level it is interesting to contemplate the influence of the residential staff member who habitually smells of smoke in a setting in which the young people are banned from smoking. In many establishments it is considered that light smoking, perhaps up to five cigarettes a day, is less than some of the other potential evils. Furthermore, adolescents are bound to flex their muscles against the rules and it may be considered better to bend the no smoking rule than many of the other regulations. This argument can of course be countered by the fact that smoking can be addictive, more so than certain drugs, and is closely related to a wide range of severe health problems in youth and particularly in later life. Is it better to turn a blind eye to minor indulgence, to have the most decrepit area in the establishment set aside for smokers or to impose severe measures on anybody caught smoking? For many young people, the problem is compounded by the fact that they were already smokers before they arrived in residence and they may be in a smoking environment during holiday periods.

For a young person who is addicted to drugs before entry or who becomes addicted during residence, the problems can be potentially greater. No residential or care establishment is likely to condone drug taking and regular testing is now common in all settings. The question arises: Should any young person who is caught either consuming or selling drugs be excluded, temporarily or permanently, or be put on an in-house or external rehabilitation programme? If the habit was learned within the establishment, it would be reasonable to suppose that there is some responsibility to help the young person towards rehabilitation.

A further health issue concerns sexual relationships in mixed and in single-sex settings. The age for consent is a matter of law and the law must be applied inside as much as it is outside. Among the adolescent population of the UK as a whole the incidents of sexually transmitted diseases is growing at an alarming rate and there is some evidence that the situation is replicated in residential settings. The problems for residential staff range from moral issues such as chastity to major health matters concerning long-term fertility. What is the potential effect upon the behaviour of the young people of a residential member of staff who constantly changes partners?

A number of principles may be applied in discussing issues of sexuality (Kahan, 1994):

- young people have a need for information and education on the issues;
- staff have a duty to discuss the issues with young people who ask for advice or help;
- staff should discuss and agree with those who have parental responsibility and the establishment who is to take responsibility for the young person's sex education;
- young people should be encouraged to feel positively responsible for their sexuality and sexual identity;
- there should be clear and understood ground rules about sexuality within residential and boarding settings.

Alcohol abuse is a serious concern in certain of the more open settings such as FE colleges, military training establishments and boarding schools. In general terms, the incidence can probably be related to the amount of time the young people are given unsupervised away from the immediate vicinity of the establishment and to the level of responsibility shown by local publicans and off-licence owners. In settings in which visits are carefully monitored and controlled, the possibility of obtaining alcohol is of course limited. However, holiday periods may well be periods of indulgence. Should limited, responsible consumption of alcohol be part of the PSHCE programme? For some young people who are genetically highly predisposed towards alcoholism, even an introduction to alcohol may be fatal, while for most it is likely to remain a pleasant addition to a meal or to life in general. In the UK, as opposed to much of the rest of Europe and the world, drunkenness is a condition to which the peer group appears to attach some form of heroic status. Therefore, the issue for residential staff is not merely one of over-indulgence and the possible long-term effects but one with many cultural and status overlays. This point again underlines the distinction between the purely medical approach and that of the residential staff.

A further issue of increasing concern is eating disorders which, while they occur predominantly among female young people, also affect a significant number of males. The increasing obesity of UK society has received a high public profile and the issue of binge eating has been raised. This is now recognised as a disorder. However, the more common problems occur with anorexia nervosa and bulimia nervosa. Although, in each case, the focus is food, the problem is emotional. Anorexia in particular is linked to self-esteem, the intention being through a restriction on eating to control body weight and shape. Gradually, the view of the person as to what is an appropriate weight and shape becomes distorted. Bulimia involves binge eating and subsequent purging through vomiting, the use of laxatives or exercise. Therefore, anorexia is more obvious to the observer than bulimia which may not result in obvious weight loss.

Both eating disorders can occur from late adolescence onwards and can be related to a lack of self-confidence, low self-esteem, various types of stress, grief, abuse or difficult relationships.

The main signs are, for anorexia, weight loss or failure to gain weight, dizziness, and for women loss of menstrual periods. For bulimia the main piece of evidence is likely to be that young people disappear after meals to vomit. The other main clue is binge eating. For both there are also emotional signs and these, together with the behavioural indicators, are discussed in Mickleburgh (2001).

In residential and boarding education and care, the occurrence of eating disorders can affect not only the individual but also the peer group and perhaps the entire community. Young people who are afflicted can become antisocial and may even indulge in the various forms of contemporary hazard. Their main requirement is for support and understanding. It is also important to be able to provide information not only about the disorders themselves but also the different approaches to treatment. All residential staff should be aware of the signs and symptoms so that treatment may be provided at an early stage. When the disorders are apparent, it is as well to seek external expertise but it is also important to develop a small internal team so that the matter is kept under constant review. As with so many medical issues, there will also be the issue of confidentiality. For residential staff not directly involved in the eating disorder team, the main points are vigilance, support, confidentiality and pastoral care.

The residential staff member is not only a model but also a guide in helping young people appreciate the importance of adopting a healthy lifestyle. The pastoral role merges education, care and health. If there is to be a serious discussion on health issues and particularly contemporary hazards, then it is vital that the residential staff have accurate and reliable information. A staff member who appears uninformed and naïve compared with the young people is unlikely to be effective.

Another role of the staff is in safeguarding the health security of the young people. For normal activities this involves a risk assessment with a major accent upon the potential health and medical problems, for which a comprehensive medical textbook should be available (e.g. Long, 2000; Smith, 2000). On the medical front, the aim is to have sufficient knowledge to know when to call for advice. The timing is likely to be more obvious in the case of physical than of mental illness. Given the rapidity and range of physical, mental, emotional and spiritual change during adolescence, it is at least as important to watch for evidence of self-harming or depression as for skin rashes. However, the major component of medical safety for most young people will concern contemporary hazards.

The law, procedures and policies of the establishment and the location of support experts and organisations should be known and understood. In particular, there needs to be an understanding of medical confidentiality, which can result in misunderstandings between medical staff, the establishment and parents or those with parental responsibility. Medical staff have a professional obligation to keep medical information about young people confidential. However, in the interests of providing care for a young person, there may be occasions where such information, if at all possible with the young person's consent, may be passed on to appropriate members of staff or parents. In such cases, should the young person refuse consent, the medical staff may still divulge it if they judge that such an action is in the interests of the young person or the establishment as a whole. As far as possible, medical staff will seek the young person's consent, anonymise the data where necessary and reduce all disclosures to a minimum. These and related points are fully discussed by Harrington (2001). There is also a list of situations in which confidential information may be disclosed to a third party. These include:

- when as a result of an emergency the young person's consent cannot be obtained;
- when it is considered to be in the young person's medical interests;

- when it is believed that the young person is a victim of abuse;
- when it is judged to be in the public interest.

Apart from general medication and treatment, confidentiality is also likely to arise in the context of contemporary hazards, particularly those concerned with sexual relationships. Guidelines have been promulgated by the Medical Officers of Schools' Association (Harrington, 2001), and these may be summarised as follows:

- doctors should be prepared to offer contraceptive advice and, when appropriate, contraception, to any young person of any age;
- contraception should be provided only after full and adequate counselling and discussion with the young person;
- young people should be encouraged to discuss contraceptive matters with their parents or those with delegated parental responsibility;
- the duty of confidentiality is owed by the doctor as in other aspects of medical practice.

Emergencies are discussed more within the field of care and welfare but those which involve health or medical conditions may be sudden and critical. As with so many aspects of residential work, time spent considering the possibilities and particularly the potential worst cases and the appropriate measures to be taken is never wasted. The most effective practitioner will be the one who is thoughtful and well prepared.

Component 3: Care and welfare

Care and welfare is the core area within which the residential staff member operates (Jack, 1998). Care includes all aspects of primary caring together with safety and overall security. It is therefore the most fundamental of the provisions offered in residence, which is why residential staff can enjoy a closer relationship with the young people than the teacher or the health professional. The residential staff stand, officially or unofficially, *in loco parentis* in that the attempt is made to replicate the best aspects of care as practised by a loving and supportive family. While it is hoped that there is some affection, esteem and at least respect in a relationship between the staff member and a young person, the level of affection found in well functioning families cannot, for obvious reasons, be replicated. The underpinning bond in the house, community or unit must be belonging, fairness and justice rather than affection (Robinson, 1994).

Primary care is the first priority and this is followed by welfare, which includes all aspects of pastoral care. Once food, clothing, shelter, basic care, safety and a healthy environment have been provided, all things being equal, the young person can complete the rite of passage and integrate with the establishment. Welfare focuses on the maintenance of a healthy and happy lifestyle as a member of the community.

It is interesting to compare the rights of the child as set out in the International Convention and the needs of children as catalogued in numerous publications. Rights cover the fundamentals and coincide with needs at a basic level. However, once the stage of self-realisation (Maslow, 1943) is reached, needs continue but rights have been fulfilled. At that stage, welfare becomes more important than care in the residential staff member's role. The higher reaches of needs, coinciding with and extending beyond welfare, are covered in PSD. Care and welfare progresses in terms defined by Maier (1987) from dependency to interdependency and finally independency.

However, such changes can only occur once the fundamentals of care including safety and a sense of belonging have been met. This sense of security within the human environment is assisted by aspects of the physical environment and the external environment. In considerations of human territoriality the focus is upon the bed space. In psychological terms, the bed space when one is asleep represents one's place of greatest security at a time of greatest vulnerability. Other personal space may be allied to the bed space such as a room or a share of a more public space. The personalisation of the bed space (FitzGerald, 1994) is therefore not merely an expression of artistic licence but a psychological need. Within reason, young people should be encouraged to bring personal belongings and momentoes to provide support for their rites of passage into and transition through the residential setting.

In many establishments such as hospitals, special schools, military training establishments and boarding schools there may be a dormitory or shared sleeping area, in which case the scope for personalisation is limited to adjacent walls and personal furniture. Whatever the available space for posters, an important aspect is the suitability of the depictions. It seems sensible that a balance be struck between artwork which illustrates the interests of the individual involved and that which, without being prudish, may be considered offensive. It is certainly an interesting lesson for residential life that one young person's rights may offend the rights of a peer or a member of staff.

The time spent on primary caring will vary according to the age group and the character of the setting. For example, in most health settings it is likely to be more dominant than in those which specialise in education. In a different way, since it may have been lacking, possibly to a marked degree before entry, care is crucial in social and, in particular, custodial settings. Many of the young people will require support initially in self-care and many of the basics of living in groups.

To feel a sense of belonging, the young person must have completed the rite of passage into the establishment and must have returned to something like the state of personal balance enjoyed before entry. Until such integration has occurred, behaviour is likely to include the atypical. Once established, the peer group becomes of particular importance. In any residential setting there will be a variety of groups but broadly speaking within a unit there will be an in-group and an out-group. Residential staff need to watch for isolates who, without group support, can suffer in all facets of development (Callow, 1994). Some young people will never be part of the in-group because they lack the cultural currency which provides status within the establishment. However, with the help of the residential staff they can develop hobbies, skills or interests and thereby become members of at least subsidiary groups. An important question which arises in this connection concerns assimilation. To what extent should young people be encouraged to retain and take a pride in their native culture and how much should they be guided towards incorporation into British culture? It is important to be able to celebrate diversity but without social fragmentation.

All staff should have a place in the pastoral system but residential staff have a more explicitly defined role, with direct responsibility for the general well-being of the young people. The fundamental needs identified in a welfare audit may have to be addressed, but the focus is upon the daily fluctuations of life rather than the major oscillations. In this, pastoral care may be compared with counselling, a specialised profession, in which more deep-seated anxieties are addressed. Apart from regular meetings and one-to-one discussions, pastoral care comprises essentially maintaining a friendly level of contact and support for the young people. The welfare audit will vary from setting to setting but is likely to be based upon the applicable National Minimum Standards, supplemented by lists of general needs (e.g. Kahan, 1994).

The welfare audit relates directly to the Care Plan which may be envisaged in two contexts. For all young people in residence there should be a basic Care Plan involving all developmental components and culled from records and staff meetings. The result is not an official document but essentially a guide for all aspects of the residential or boarding care of the young person. It should be proactive in setting out the aims for each aspect and constructed taking advice from all relevant sources including the young person and, if appropriate, the family. In the case of young people looked after by local authorities and other agencies, the Care Plan is an official document in which clearly stated objectives are set out for care together with a strategy for achieving these objectives. It is constructed so that all participants understand the role that residential care will play in meeting the young person's overall needs. The decision to change such a Care Plan may only be made at a statutory review. For constructing a Care Plan there are several key sources (e.g. DoH, 2000a, 2000b; Iwaniec and Hill, 1999). The following dimensions are basic:

- identity;
- health;
- education;
- social presentation;
- self-care;

- social and personal relationships;
- emotional and behavioural development.

All staff need to be aware of the policies and procedures of the establishment so that advice given to the young people is within the appropriate guidelines. With thought, application, a good sense of self-awareness (Hutchinson, 1994) and real interest in young people, any member of staff is capable of becoming an effective pastoral carer.

While counselling is a specialised role requiring specific training, underlying skills, such as active listening and providing evidence of interest and attention while the young person is talking, can be practised by all residential staff. As far as is sensible, the power differential between the staff member and the young person needs to be reduced so that an empathetic working relationship may be established. If no such relationship seems possible, it is probably preferable to transfer the young person to another pastoral group (Hutchinson, 1993).

Counselling skills would normally be deployed in a face-to-face discussion with a young person in the context of relatively serious problems. Since the situation is necessarily one of intimacy, the staff member must take into account the child protection issues. For productive counselling the following core conditions are likely to obtain:

- there will be empathy;
- there will be mutual respect;
- there will be a feeling of genuineness in the relationship;
- there will be sufficient self-knowledge so that the young person can be helped;
- there will be congruence between the verbal exchanges and the body language;
- there will be immediacy and an incisive approach.

(Eggert, 1999)

In the same volume, one particular aspect of great relevance, bereavement counselling is also discussed. The most likely meeting of death for the young person is when a parent or close relative dies. Staff who are present at the time need to offer reassurance, the opportunity to talk and a quiet place for contemplation. Those who are bereaved normally go through a number of stages and the whole process may take up to two years. Recognised stages include:

- denial in which reality cannot be accepted;
- emotion, frequently expressed as anger;
- guilt that more support should have been given to the person who has died;
- fantasy when reality is replaced by some other outcome;
- helplessness which needs to be addressed by coping skills;

- depression which can influence all aspects of life;
- acceptance when the feeling of loss has become manageable.

The staff pastoral role may also involve advocacy, providing active support normally in verbal form for the young people. Advocacy may be required as part of the complaints procedure since one of the key features of the *Children Act* (1989) is that no young person living in an ex-familial setting should feel cut off from advice and support. Such support may also come from visitors or members of the peer group. If young people are to have greater control over their destinies then, in many cases, they will need the empowerment which advocacy can bring. Closely related to advocacy is negotiation which implies the attainment of a settlement or agreement through consultation and conferring. The two terms are linked in a systems approach discussed by Coulshed and Orme (1998).

Pastoral work may be informal as happens, for example, in children's homes and many small group settings where every member of staff has pastoral duties. In boarding schools, special schools, military establishments and FE colleges there is likely to be a designated member of staff, a divisional officer or a moral tutor who acts on pastoral matters for a small group of the young people. There may also be set times for pastoral activities, although it is realised that need may not coincide with the preferred programme. In general, the larger the establishment the more elaborate the pastoral structure has to be and the greater the difficulty in ensuring that every troubled young person has a well-defined route to seeking advice.

The pastoral role may not comprise solely waiting for a young person to bring a problem. The residential staff also need to be proactive to intervene as appropriate. The judgement as to whether or when to intervene is among the most subtle to be made by residential staff (Aguilera, 1994). When should the situation be allowed to run and when has deterioration reached the point where intervention is needed? The answer of course depends upon the situation but particularly upon a thorough knowledge of the young people involved. It may also vary considerably according to the setting, since, for example, young people in an FE college are likely to consider themselves to be relatively self-sufficient. In general, there is more scope for error in timing in FE colleges, boarding schools and children's homes than in custodial settings. The most effective residential staff are those who have thought carefully about potential problems and appropriate interventions before they are faced with the reality.

Care and welfare also entails crises and emergencies and the safeguarding of the young people. The residential staff must be completely familiar with establishment policies for all likely emergencies ranging from fire and flood to the presence of an intruder or absconding (Wade and Biehal, 1998). The staff handbook and guidance must be thoroughly digested because crises are bound to occur, if very rarely, and there may be no second chance to act effectively. Apart from guidelines, it is also vital to know the location of all key controls in the establishment so that electricity, water, gas and other services may be switched off and appropriate outside services contacted. The address and telephone list of all external support, whatever the emergency, must be readily available. If there are no paper or role-playing exercises, worst case scenarios must be thought through.

A further area within care and welfare and with which the residential staff member must be familiar is special educational needs (Gabbitas Educational Consultants, 2003–2004). In familiarisation with all the records and personal details of the young people for whom there is responsibility, those with statements or other special needs will be apparent. Clearly it is appropriate that specific problems, such as epileptic fits, which may need to be addressed, require prior study. While there will be special medication as appropriate and support from medical and health professionals, the basic care remains the responsibility of the residential staff (Lishman, 1991). Particular vigilance is required with regard to the secure storage of medicines.

At the least, the residential staff should have a basic idea of special needs. The following classification is based on the Gabbitas Guide to which has been added a set of explanatory notes.

1   *Attention deficit/hyperactivity disorder (AD/HD)*: this is a developmental disorder in which young people cannot function properly in sustaining attention, controlling impulses and gearing their level of activity appropriately.
2   *Autism*: this is a developmental disability affecting communication skills. There is a spectrum of autism but all autistic people have difficulty with social interaction, communication with others and in having limited imagination.
3   *Cerebral palsy*: this is a physical impairment which affects movement. There is a spectrum ranging from barely noticeable difficulties to severe problems. In extreme cases, young people are unable to walk, feed, talk, use their hands or even sit up without help from others. Where it is obvious, cerebral palsy may be seen in lack of movement control, unwanted movements or problems with balance.
4   *Cystic fibrosis*: this is a life-threatening inherited disease which results in damage to the major organs. The most obvious effect is upon the lungs and there may also be difficulties with digestion.
5   *Down's syndrome*: this results from an accident before or at the time of conception which gives rise to the development of an extra chromosome. The result is a number of physical characteristics which affect the appearance of the young person. There are commonly problems with hearing and vision, heart defects, lack of muscle tone, and speech and language difficulties.
6   *Dyscalculia*: this is a learning difficulty which impedes the learning of mathematics and may be associated with other learning difficulties.

7 *Dyslexia*: this is a specific learning difficulty which hinders the learning of literacy skills at all levels of intellectual ability.

8 *Dyspraxia*: this is an impairment or immaturity of the organisation of movement and may be associated with language perception and thought problems. The term which may be employed is 'developmental dyspraxia' or 'developmental coordination disorder'.

9 *Epilepsy*: this is indicated by a tendency for the brain to experience recurrent seizures in which total or partial consciousness may be lost.

10 *Gifted*: the unusual or special abilities attributed to gifted young people include creativity, interest in learning and speed of learning. Approximately 2 per cent of the school population is said to be gifted. The term normally used in education is 'gifted and talented'.

11 *Hearing impairment*: few young people are totally deaf, and hearing impairment may be divided into conductive, in which a blockage prevents the sound from passing into the middle ear or to the nerve of hearing; or sensori-neural, in which the nerve of hearing does not process the sound effectively. Some young people suffer from mixed deafness when both types are present.

12 *Leukaemia*: this is a cancer of the blood, and symptoms include anaemia, problems with infection and abnormal bruising. Treatment by intensive chemotherapy and also possibly radiotherapy, together with the cancer itself, may lead to learning difficulties and a range of side effects, including emotional concerns.

13 *Limb deficiency*: this indicates birth without the whole or part of a limb, but clearly limbs may be lost as the result of an accident or amputation. Difficulties are practical and emotional, and are compounded during the process of learning to use artificial limbs (prostheses).

14 *Muscular dystrophy*: this is a general name given to several conditions in which there is a breakdown of muscle fibres, leading to weak and wasted muscles. Disability varies from severe to mild, but most of the conditions cause progressive weakening of the muscles.

15 *Speech and language difficulties*: most children with special educational needs (SEN) have speech and communication difficulties and some have specific or primary speech or language impairment.

16 *Spina bifida*: this is a developmental defect of the neural tube which occurs soon after conception. The result is that bone or vertebrae fail to form properly, leaving a gap or split. Spina bifida occulta is very mild and rarely causes disability. Spina bifida cystica, which results in a visible sac or cyst on the back, depending on its form, may result in either little disability or serious problems. In the latter case there is likely to be some degree of paralysis and loss of sensation below the damaged vertebrae. There may also be bladder and bowel control problems and a lack of mobility.

17 *Gilles de la Tourette syndrome*: this is associated with dysfunction in areas of the brain which are responsible for movement and the control of

inhibition and impulsivity. The main symptom is involuntary movement or noise known as tics, which may be simple or complex. There may also be displays of obsessive compulsive behaviour.

18 *Visual impairment*: few children are totally without sight, some can only distinguish light and dark and some have only central or peripheral vision. Many have additional disabilities or a combination of impairments.

For fuller descriptions, the *Gabbitas Guide to Schools for Special Needs* (Gabbitas Educational Consultants, 2003–2004) is recommended. For each of the disabilities listed together with gifted and talented children, there are specialist organisations which can supply further details on treatment and educational requirements. It would seem reasonable that residential staff throughout all sectors should be reasonably conversant with the special needs terminology and with the *Children Act* (1989) in relation to children with disabilities (DoH, 1991c; Read and Clements, 2001).

In all this endeavour, the residential staff member is acting as a reasonable parent and may in fact have, at certain times, delegated parental responsibility (Chapter 3). Therefore, it is important to maintain an external network which provides appropriate support for the young people. First and foremost, family contact is vital (Chakrabati and Hill, 2000). Confidence must be established between those natural parents or whoever has responsibility and the person within the establishment who has temporary pastoral responsibility. Of course, this does not mean that life within the setting should attempt to replicate that of the family. The family model may be a form of ideal but it is one which may not have been experienced by many of the young people in residence. Therefore, respect for family members does not necessarily mean acceptance of their directives. It may well be that pastoral work should be extended from the young person to the family if at the end of the period of residence there is to be an optimum chance for a happy, healthy and productive lifestyle. Familial bonds are extremely strong and every attempt needs to be made to achieve a balance, accepted by both parties, between the aims of the establishment and the requests of the family (Colton *et al.*, 2001).

Partnership with parents or those with parental responsibility is a cornerstone of the *Children Act* (1989) and, ideally, this fact should be made apparent by the provision of a handbook or at least written notes for parents, setting out relevant information including details on:

- visiting by both the young person and the parent;
- contact with the young person and key staff;
- important names and addresses;
- complaints procedure;
- pastoral care system;
- discipline and expected behaviour;
- the health and medical system;

- personal clothes/equipment allowed and pocket money;
- other aspects of the establishment considered important.

In the field of care and welfare, the residential staff member is faced with a vast range of issues and problems and the need to achieve a balanced outcome. It is often difficult to judge success which may be ultimate rather than proximate but failure may be readily indicated. The effective practitioner is distinguished as the one who is thoroughly prepared for all eventualities and has carefully thought through the sorts of problems which might arise in the lives of the young people for whom there is responsibility.

Component 4: Personal and social development

In the UK, as family life has changed, so parenting as a subject has entered schools. Schools are expected not only to fulfil something of the role of parents but also to teach many of the skills which in previous times would have been taught by parents. Initially, personal and social education was recognised as a cross-curricular topic and this has now metamorphosed into personal, social, health and citizenship education (PSHCE) (Inman *et al.*, 1998). Citizenship is essentially a specialised form of social education as a result of which social concerns should influence the behaviour of a person within a group. It relies on a number of personal qualities, for example, the desire to contribute. Therefore, it is contended that PSD, with the exception of health, covers the array of subjects included in PSHCE.

Personal development includes a wide range of characteristics, many of which are interrelated. Basic are identity and self-esteem in that without these there is little to build upon. Others include self-confidence, reliance, resilience and independence. All may be demonstrated in some behaviours and not in others. Therefore, in attempting to identify progress, it is important that as many viewpoints as possible are obtained. In general, there is a progression from selfishness, through conformity to independence. It appears that it is necessary to conform to the norms of a community or society before independence can be demonstrated (Hunt and Sullivan, 1974). Certain of the characteristics, such as self-esteem, are integral to the individual. Other personal characteristics, although they do not necessarily involve interaction, do presuppose a group setting. Among these are reliance, resilience and independence. In the context of group living, resilience may be needed to withstand the rigours of the human and physical environments. For example, in custodial settings, a move from a LASU to a YOI involves a total change of environments and, if the benefits of residence in the LASU are to be retained, such a characteristic is required (Rose, 2002). Further, it may be said that for any young person without support, leaving a residential environment will require resilience to be successful in the world outside. To address this issue, many of the settings have adopted a halfway house procedure which remains under the jurisdiction of the establishment but allows semi-independence and therefore greater responsibility before leaving.

In the classic model, personal precedes social development. Young people are supported individually before being subjected to group conditions, paralleling development within a family. In residential and boarding education and care, the reverse procedure, by necessity, occurs. The young person is put directly into a group living situation and only if there is obvious failure are the personal characteristics immediately addressed. For a young person with low self-esteem, entering a relatively large residential establishment such as an FE college, boarding school, YOI or special school, life must appear fraught and the rites of passage may extend over a long time period before a state of incorporation is reached.

It is clear that many attributes of personal development (Anderson, 1993), while being integral to the individual, can only be identified in the presence of another person. The distinction between personal and social is therefore somewhat blurred and this clearly affects the diagnosis of problems. In a simple situation, if a young person is faced with a plate of cakes and eats them all, assuming the normal life-sustaining systems were in place in the community, the characteristic might be labelled as greed. If the plate of cakes was on the table as part of the team tea, the characteristic might be more appropriately called selfish. The first is essentially personal; the second is personal but can be demonstrated only in the context of others.

With these caveats in mind, social development is seen as the way in which the individual fits into the human environment. This involves a range of relationships including those with peers, with young people of different ages and with adults. It involves a series of attributes connected with teamwork, accepting decisions and leadership. In this context, training for a team game such as football or netball can have far more significance than merely the potential to achieve sporting success.

In the full range of settings, the question might be asked as to whether integration into the group is necessarily beneficial. For example, for young people segregated as a result of social or behavioural problems, group contact may enhance the difficulties. Nonetheless, if success in later life is to be achieved, it is necessary for young people to survive in their own peer groups. For this reason, there is a general move throughout all settings to encourage more group work, group living and association. This has long been one of the lessons of boarding in which a considerable proportion of residential and even some academic education may be attributable to peers (Cowie and Wallace, 2000). Group living raises many of the issues considered in terms of the human environment.

In any group situation, it appears that a pecking order is established. This may be completely informal or formalised, it may be exact or it may represent a broad hierarchy. It is clearly vital to know, in terms of social development, how status is derived (Chapter 2). It may result from a particular talent such as sporting ability or quick-wittedness, it may relate to size and strength, it may correlate with length of stay or it may be achieved as a result of a particular action. The required orientation for the establishment is towards a position in which status is derived from a wide variety of desirable attributes and abilities. In this context, it may be seen how most boarding schools have changed over the past thirty years so that the ambience is not dominated by sporting prowess but includes music, drama, academic pursuits and a number of other characteristics.

Bullying can appear in a number of forms but physical bullying and status related to size and strength remain a dangerous combination. Logically, verbal bullying and a malicious tongue may be even more difficult in that signs of physical bullying are more likely to be overt whereas verbal bullying is likely to flourish away from any staff surveillance (DfE, 1994). Obviously, if in a custodial setting status derives from the scale of the crime committed, a total staff effort is required to change the climate.

For residential staff, the PSD of the young people is a key consideration. As discussed, it relates closely to the other developmental areas and a case can be made that it is the single most important component of development. However, it is the least formalised and the most difficult to assess. Ideally, PSD should be a concern of all staff and, in this, it is different from the other four developmental components, in which all the staff may well be interested but not all will play a direct part. Of particular relevance are the domestic staff. The matron or a matron-like figure has long been important in residential living in special schools and boarding schools. Apart from primary caring, the matron can act as a supportive figure to whom the young people can relate. She, or possibly he, can offer uncritical comfort to the young people and, without betraying confidences, supply crucial information related to PSD to the residential staff. Other familiar figures such as cooks and cleaners also have a role in that they are likely to have a special position in the lives of the young people and a unique viewpoint from which to assess PSD. They, possibly more than any other members of staff, can remain in the confidence of both the young people and the staff while offering assistance to both. Their viewpoint is quite different from that of residential staff in that they are far more likely to see the young people in unguarded moments, and in fact of all staff, they approach closest to 'street life'. For example, bad behaviour, at least in its milder forms, such as swearing, may not stop in their presence whereas it probably would cease if a member of the residential staff appeared.

In view of these considerations, it is essential that all members of staff are familiar with the PSD aims of the setting. If they do not know what is expected, they are unlikely to be able to offer appropriate assistance. The philosophy, aims and ethos of each establishment will be to an extent unique but are likely to include reference to the five developmental components identified. In the case of PSD, an increasingly relevant question is whether the aims of the establishment accord with those of society at large. This question of course faces all schools but is particularly pertinent in the more controlled environment of residence. One answer is that, as the values of society are changing and becoming somewhat opaque, the establishment should attempt to inculcate those, such as honesty and truth, which are timeless.

An interesting distinction is that between proximate and ultimate aims. How much should the establishment concern itself with what can be achieved during the term of residence and how much should be directed at later life? As discussed (Chapter 3), the aim is to prepare young people for life and therefore skills which last a lifetime must be important. However, with the advent of Standards and inspections, the establishment will be judged upon what it achieves during residence.

If the family is the setting in which most young people develop personally and socially, should this be the model for residential living? It is frequently mentioned as a truism that families are the best places for the upbringing of young people. However, in the UK today in the light of the variety and number of less than fully functioning families, this statement bears at least some discussion (Chapter 2). Some family homes provide what is a very difficult environment, virtually inimical to the development of young people. This may have little or nothing to do with choice and may be related to any number of social characteristics ranging from poverty to neglect or criminality.

As a result, for some young people a residential setting must be preferable to either family life or fostering. Apart from potential child protection risks, theoretically greater in fostering than residence, the intensity of a family lifestyle without the natural parents does not suit some young people. Therefore, residential and boarding education and care may be the best choice. The only community which can supply undemanding love is the family, and the lack of such love for the period of residence, depending upon its length and particularly its continuity, is clearly something of a negative factor. On the other hand, such love may not be proffered, in which case the respect and support of the residence may provide at least a partial substitute.

For social development, the residential environment has obvious benefits. In most modern families there are few children and they vary in age. In residential settings, there are likely to be several members of the same age group as well as some who are older and some who are younger. Therefore, the family profile age-wise is maintained and there is a far larger peer group within which social development can take place. For single-child families, opportunities for social development are obviously limited through the lack of peers in the living environment. For young people, both of whose parents are largely absentees through the pressures of long working days, there may be little parental contribution to social education. Therefore, while in no way disparaging the importance of the family in the development of the young people, it is possible to see that residential experience can provide opportunities which are otherwise denied to them. Single-child families or families in which both parents are largely absentees through workload may offer little in the way of social education. In residence, there is always the peer group in which social skills will be developed.

As with other developmental components, it is possible to construct a chronological profile for the progress of each young person. This would tend to follow the threefold division of dependent, conforming and independent. However, there are many attributes which may be examined in order to establish dependency and the answers derived may not coincide. It is possible to be independent in one personal attribute but dependent in another. Some young people will enter the setting at a later stage on a particular scale than others. Therefore, an assessment of PSD poses an array of problems and is, as a result, commonly addressed in only the most superficial way. In reports, there may be comments about relationships with adults or self-presentation but normally little evidence is provided and the characteristics in question are rarely set in the totality of PSD. Furthermore, from the scientific viewpoint, since all the young people are, broadly speaking, within the same environment, it is not possible to have any form of control group. For the other four components there are norms, in some cases national norms which can be invoked. For PSD any evidence is likely to be qualitative rather than quantitative and judgements are made in comparison with what is considered normal in the establishment.

Some problems of assessment may be overcome if all members of staff involved with a particular young person are included in the monitoring procedure. This presupposes that all have been involved in the identification and definition of the aims of PSD. The effect of this is not only that there is a wide range of inputs and everyone is aware of the establishment's mission but that a reasonable measure of validity is obtained through replication and all staff have ownership of the system. If staff views are collected on agreed rating scales at regular intervals, the problems of reliability and validity are considerably lessened, if not overcome, by the degree of replication. For example, if twenty-five of the thirty staff members agree on a particular point, this shows a higher degree of certainty than is evident in most aspects of social science. In addition, the points raised by the remaining five can be examined and may, as a result of a differing viewpoint, add considerably to the knowledge about the young person. At the very least, regular staff meetings to consider each child or young person must be beneficial and must facilitate the identification of problems. It is then possible to focus the attention of residential staff upon particular young people and specific issues (Anderson, 1993).

Component 5: Behaviour

In residential living, behaviour is considered in two contexts. Behaviour, in a scientific context, is taken to indicate evidence of change, most obvious in PSD. It is possible to identify the acquisition of certain personal or social attributes as a result of behaviour. In discussing behaviour as a development component, the term is related to the type and quality of behaviour and in particular how it affects other people within the setting. For example, the behaviour during a fire practice or actual fire is an absolute, with no negotiation possible. Behaviour in its everyday context may be considered good or bad or anything in between. According to the philosophy of the establishment, it may be unwanted or antisocial. There is a spectrum of behaviour from, say, poor table manners, which may be unpleasant and unacceptable, to violent and challenging activity. Furthermore, distressing behaviour may be self-directed, possibly in the form of self-mutilation, rather than necessarily projected against other people.

A code of conduct might cover the following:

- bad language;
- politeness;
- punctuality;
- quietness;
- tidiness;
- respect for the fabric of the establishment and the property of other people;
- stealing;
- smoking;
- the use of alcohol, illegal drugs and solvents;
- cleanliness and neatness of appearance;
- the wearing of particular adornments;
- bounds and appropriate arrival and leaving procedures.

For any setting, there is likely to be a normal range of acceptable behaviour. Anything beyond that range may attract a response varying from a reproach to a sanction to attempts at behaviour modification. Since behaviour is the outward sign of a variety of internal and external factors, it is scarcely surprising that during adolescence behaviour is inconsistent (Varma, 1997). During the passage into and out of the establishment, atypical and possibly deviant behaviour is likely to occur. Such behaviour may also be related to regular events such as getting up, going to bed or at weekends. For the establishment the aim is, as far as possible, to inculcate what is taken to be normal behaviour and to encourage the young people in self-regulation. For example, if behavioural change is only brought about by sanctions, what will happen when controls are removed when the young person leaves residence?

In all settings, behaviour ranging from the unwanted to the challenging is likely to be faced at some time. Therefore, members of staff need to be fully aware of what is acceptable behaviour by the young people and also the staff response when such behaviour does not occur. This may take the form of a tariff of rewards and sanctions for clearly defined behaviours or it may be more broadly based, relying largely upon the discretion of the residential staff. In either case, risk must be taken into account and an attempt made to achieve a balance between reasonable order or discipline and a free environment in which the young people are encouraged to express themselves and to make their own decisions.

Certain types of behaviour are considered so insidious that they attract their own establishment policy. The most obvious among these are bullying and abuse. Bullying is probably endemic in any group and, in a group of young people living through the changes and chances of adolescence, it is unlikely to be totally eradicated. Physical bullying can be shown to be so much against the ambience of the establishment that it does not occur but verbal bullying is far more difficult to control. Indeed, since verbal bullying grades into being unkind or unfriendly, it is difficult to define and therefore poses problems for staff intervention. The most positive approach for residential staff is to help develop a shared concern throughout the community for any cases of bullying and, in many establishments, the adoption of a no-blame policy has been effective (Sharp and Smith, 1994).

There is no precise definition of bullying but there are common elements in such behaviour which can be recognised. It occurs when some form of harassment goes beyond a certain threshold and it may be seen in all walks of life. However, the opportunity is particularly great among young people living away from home in groups. The main points about bullying are:

- it is persistent and involves repeated events;
- it is perpetrated by an individual or group against someone perceived as in some way weaker;
- it is deliberate and intended to result in some form of domination.

Bullying may be physical or verbal, or involve extortion or exclusion from social groups or activities. It is particularly insidious because it can be very subtle and dominate the life of the victim. Furthermore, bullying is likely to occur in places and at times when it is most inaccessible to staff. Given its covert nature, it is vital that residential staff remain sensitive and vigilant at all times. The effect on the victim may range from unhappiness to depression and even the contemplation of suicide, and the effects of bullying are likely at least to inhibit development. Sadly, even in the best-run settings it is unlikely that bullying will be eliminated altogether.

Residential staff should be thoroughly conversant with the anti-bullying policy of the establishment and how it should be implemented. The policy itself will include aims, a definition of bullying, an inventory of preventive measures and procedures to be followed when an incident occurs. For every incident, a full record is required, and this will include:

- the names of those involved;
- the time and place of the incident;
- characteristics of the incident;

- action taken;
- follow-up action.

If there is an obvious shared concern about bullying among all staff and young people, the number of incidents will be minimised.

Abuse has been covered in detail (Chapter 3) but suffice it to say that emotional abuse and verbal bullying may well be indistinguishable. Indeed, abuse constitutes a specialised form of bullying in that it represents the oppression of the less powerful by the more powerful. This again brings into question the issue of status and the cultural currency of size and strength among the young people.

Violent behaviour may vary from minor damage to the fabric to severe personal injury. It is the responsibility of the residential staff to prevent any young person from causing damage which is personal, to other members of the community or to the environment. In monitoring the young people and their behaviour, those with a low threshold for violence may be identified and the conditions which set off the cycle of violence addressed (Faupel *et al.*, 1998). Violence and conflict are obviously closely related and, through careful monitoring, sources of conflict may be reduced or eliminated (Brady, 1993).

However, this requires skilled practice, professionally authoritative oversight and strong internal and external management as well as considerable commitment from the individual staff concerned (Kahan, 1994). The extremes which staff may have to face include young people who have committed serious crimes or young people on remand who are preoccupied with a delinquent crisis of offending. Other young people may experience complex self-destructive urges and some may have disturbing behaviour yet to be properly diagnosed.

When violence or conflict appears imminent or has occurred, it may well be necessary for residential staff to use physical restraint. It is essential that all staff liable to find themselves in the position of confronting violence or conflict know exactly the policy and procedures of the establishment and to be well practised in the forms of restraint used. There should be procedures clearly set out so that the young people are prevented from damaging themselves, each other, members of staff or the establishment. Physical intervention is justified in the short term to assist the young person to gain control and in the longer term to help the young person learn to cope with problems. It is defined as the use of physical force by one or more members of staff that limits or totally restricts the ability of the young person to move. The accent should be on care so that there should be the minimum use of force to achieve the goal of de-escalating the situation. Before attempting physical restraint it is important that the following criteria are met:

- that physical restraint is accepted within the policy framework of the establishment;
- that the staff member has knowledge of the correct procedure;

- that physical control is appropriate for the young person;
- that physical control is appropriate for the situation.

The most common situation in which physical intervention is required is when there is an altercation or fight between two young people. If there are not two members of staff present, then the single member needs to assess carefully the potential for making a successful physical restraint. However, physical restraint is always a traumatic experience for both staff and young people and it is vital that there is a calm therapeutic discussion session afterwards. All such cases of restraint should be recorded in detail and should form part of a report to senior management. No member of staff should ever attempt physical restraint unless the techniques are well known and have been practised.

At a lesser level, conflict resolution grades into counselling and pastoral care. The residential staff member is in a favourable position to act as mediator or to conduct negotiations between the disputants so that honour is settled and no blame attached. Ideally, the establishment will have a system which recognises the importance of conflict diffusion and that all staff are aware of the ways in which this may be achieved.

For each young person, it is possible to construct a profile of baseline behaviour so that any deviation may be seen in the context of the individual rather than the group. Remedial action may then be taken through pastoral care, counselling, conflict resolution or behaviour modification. Most residential staff are not trained in behaviour modification and, although the basic ideas are relatively straightforward, external expertise is normally required, at least to set up the procedures. The basis for behaviour modification techniques which are likely to be applicable in residential and boarding education and care is rewarding, in some form, good behaviour so that it becomes the norm (Cigno and Bourn, 1998). This type of approach comes within the realm of behavioural psychology. In cognitive psychology an attempt is made to produce positive behavioural change by discussion so that alternative interpretations or choices may be made. A further measure is provided by analytical psychology, practised by psychotherapists or counsellors. As an example of this, the young person's unwanted behaviour may be interpreted in the context of life experiences and significant relationships. Kahan (1994) discusses these schools of thought and the possible use of an eclectic approach.

An important issue is how behaviours are defined. In the clinical approach discrete problems are identified and an attempt is made to provide a remedy for each. This medical model is described in detail by Hoghughi (1980) who sets out the following categories:

- physical problems;
- intellectual and educational problems;

- home and family problems;
- social skills problems;
- antisocial behaviour problems;
- personal problems.

When backed by clear definitions, such a classification does allow the identification of recognisable situations and behaviours which may then be addressed. The main criticism is that each category need not necessarily be considered individually as a change of regime may alleviate several categories simultaneously. Psychology models tend to take a more broadly based approach in the identification and treatment of fundamental difficulties which themselves encompass a range of problems. For example, 'acting out' may be seen as a problem in itself or as a symptom of some more general underlying condition. If that condition can be modified, then the 'acting out' together with a variety of other problems may be reduced or eliminated.

In custodial care settings, there are likely to be more specialised forms of approach to behaviour (Hollin *et al.*, 1995), based upon the ideas of cognitive psychology. For example, a great deal of violent behaviour results from reflex actions. If the young people can be encouraged to adopt a more introspective approach and think for a few moments, a more rational behaviour than violence may come to mind. Philosophy courses in which logical thinking and critical reasoning (Thomson, 2002) are developed can help young people realise the variety of rationales available in any given situation. It is also important, not only in custodial settings, that young people confront their offending behaviour if rehabilitation is to be effective.

To this may be added approaches such as restorative justice (Pitts, 1999). Since both the victim and the community have been harmed, restoration is needed. In the search not only for restoration but also for prevention, the procedure includes all those who have been in any way negatively affected by the offence. The effect is that the young person should become aware of the full extent of the misbehaviour and this awareness then forms the starting point for a pastoral or therapeutic programme which is focused on the individual but owned by all the participants. However, these are all specialised procedures for which there are guidelines, and the residential staff will normally be expected to support such approaches and possibly to provide evidence but not to be a key initiator.

A particularly important staff role with regard to behaviour is monitoring and assessment. In all settings, behaviours of individuals need to be observed and deviance or something obviously atypical noted. Full reports on behaviour during daily living allow the construction of effective Care Plans. Attached to the Care Plan may be some form of contract, an idea well established in special schools and gaining currency throughout residence. Rather than sanctions for specified behaviour, the young person enters into a contract which indicates the concomitants of behaving in a particular fashion.

Antisocial behaviour can threaten the security of all members of the community and therefore needs to be addressed effectively and rapidly. As with all developmental components, the thoughtful practitioner will have considered, in the light of the young people for whom there is responsibility, possible worst case scenarios and how these might be addressed.

Chapter 5

Time components

Time as a key factor in residential and boarding education and care has already been introduced in the context of the developmental components. The interaction of the environmental and framework components summarises the operation of the particular setting at any moment in time. This may be represented as daily living. The longer term effects upon the young people are encapsulated in the developmental components, a synopsis of which is represented by transitions (Figure 5.1). The time components therefore provide a completely different viewpoint for the consideration of residential and boarding life.

In many families, given all the changes which result from modern living, less time is spent with the children than perhaps twenty or thirty years ago. The opportunities for living and learning have been greatly reduced and in some dysfunctional families virtually eliminated. Parenting by families is under strain and schools have had to help provide a solution. Clearly the role of parents as partners with the school in bringing up young people has become less clear-cut. Despite these increasing burdens, the day school has to try and cover the full academic, cultural and sporting programme within, at best, about seven hours per day for five days a week. To perform much the same task, the residential establishment with education on the premises has effectively twice the number of hours per day together with, in many cases, weekends. If, as with most children's homes the school is external, there is still likely to be more time for parenting activities than obtains commonly in families. In particular, in all forms of residence there is the invaluable informal time with staff and peer group when residential or boarding education occurs. With at most two siblings as the family norm, the case could be made that there are more opportunities for enhanced social development in residence than in the family.

Length of stay

While, in residential settings as opposed to day schools, there is potentially more time for learning and development, this is obviously conditioned by the length of stay of the young people. This raises a number of interesting issues. All things being equal, what is the minimum time in which residential living

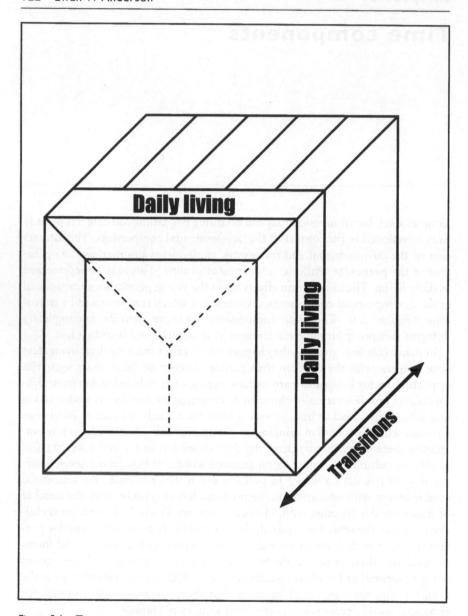

Figure 5.1   Time components

can be expected to have any effect? Do the effects vary from setting to setting? In general terms, boarding provides the extremes on the time scale. Residence is normally longer, often considerably longer if preparatory schools are taken into account, than in other sectors. The differences are so great that it is impossible to give meaningful averages but placements concerned with social factors –

children's homes, some special schools, therapeutic communities and secure units – vary from months or even weeks to one or two years. In STCs the average stay is between two months and about one year. In YOIs, whatever the sentence, since the entry age is 16, two years is the maximum period of residence for the age group under consideration. There may be relatively long-stay young people in psychiatric units, hospital schools and some special schools but average length of stay in the health sector still falls well short of that in boarding schools. The obvious exceptions would be the special schools dealing with the following: sensory and/or physical disabilities, and communication and interaction disabilities. In some of these special schools, young people may have a full educational career matching in length that in a boarding school. However, in the secondary stage of education such young people constitute well under 10 per cent of all the long-stay children in residential and boarding education and care (Figure 5.2).

Thus there are major differences according to the sector and setting in length of stay. However, some boarding schools also include different categories of residents: weekly boarders and flexi-boarders. Weekly boarders, who go home at weekends, provide an interesting category in that their style of residence may represent potentially the most effective of partnerships between residence and parents. For weekly boarders, is their 'home' within the school or with their parents? In other settings, the length of stay is normally continuous for at least a month or two. It is clear in such cases that the young person must be committed to the residential establishment. Is it the same with weekly boarding? Flexi-boarding, namely staying for the occasional night, provides at best a sub-liminal look at residential education. The bed space of flexi-boarders is at their parental home and therefore they do not have the clear-cut commitment to residence.

Continuity of time

This discussion raises a number of points about the continuity of residence. For the majority of young people – all those in FE colleges, military training establishments and boarding schools, the majority in special schools and some in health settings – there will be times away from the establishment in terms of weekends, half-terms or holidays. For those in custodial care, together with some young people in the health and social sectors there are, for differing reasons, few if any periods spent away from the establishment. This distinction emphasises the differing problems of attempting to establish and maintain partnership with parents.

The question must be asked in the context of personal and social development: Can a relatively short but continuous period of residence be more effective than a considerably longer but interrupted period? If continuity is important, what is the minimum period in which effective work can be done? In general terms, the custodial, health and social sectors tend to have longer

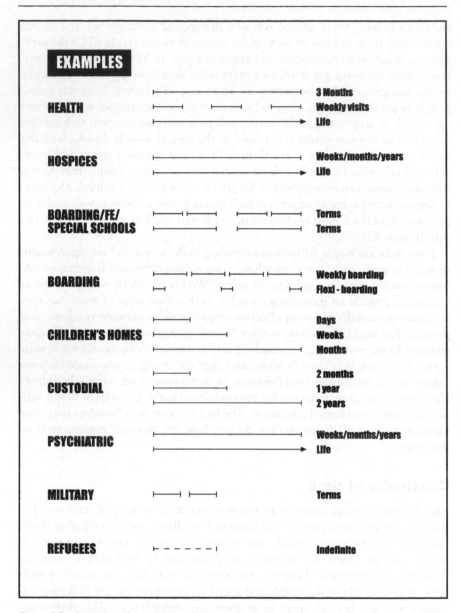

Figure 5.2   Length and continuity of time

continuous periods of residence than the educational sector. Some special schools have a pattern of terms and visits that corresponds with that in boarding schools. In boarding and some special schools, the young people visit their parents and families on a regular basis. In the custodial, and many of the health and social settings, there are meetings only if the families visit the young people.

This raises the question of the influence of family contacts on personal and social development (Hill, 1999).

In custodial and specialist health or social settings, there are comparatively few establishments and therefore catchments are usually large. As a result, distance is a key factor in limiting family contact. Distance also results in a lack of support from the establishment once the young person's period of residence has ended. This can well prove an issue for all types of setting but for those leaving custodial care there will be particular problems, as they will be unlikely to have pre-existing close links with local YOTs or probation and other services. With interrupted periods of residence, family time is possible but this is not the case with continuous residence. This introduces the question of whether continuity of residence, allowing more time for personal and social development, can compensate for more frequent family contacts. The weekly boarder who sleeps in the school for only five nights a week can have more of a family life than the boarder who goes home only once during the term. However, the latter benefits from boarding education, the bulk of which is likely to occur during weekends.

With or without the overt support of families it is important that, apart from formal education, medical care and any specialist treatment, young people can benefit from residential education. It is generally accepted, although there is little evaluative research, that to develop personally and as a member of a team a period of residence is a favoured option. The deliberate choice of residence is reflected in the development of normal child care practice. For example, intermediate treatment was introduced in many forms but a basic pattern was that the young person spent the week in day school and the weekend away in residence. Enrichment courses of various kinds for young people are frequently residential since this provides not only a social experience but also total immersion in the subject. Therefore, if a young person is to spend only two months in an STC, it must be assumed that some residential education benefit is possible.

A further interesting point arises from the fact that, with the few exceptions where lifetime incarceration is involved, boarding is likely to be by some distance the major long-term component of the system. The effects and particularly benefits of residence are best, initially at least, investigated in boarding schools. It is a basic contention of this book that the major issues in residential and boarding education and care are generic, and this fact should allow some beneficial transfer of ideas and practice between settings.

The length of residence must also be seen in the context of what is achieved during the time. For some young people the aim can be realised in a relatively short time period. For example, a limited period in a hospital school may result in a cure. In a special school a learning difficulty may be sufficiently overcome or a type of behaviour adequately controlled for the young person to return to mainstream schooling within a reasonably short space of time. In the case of boarding, residence in years twelve and thirteen only may be undertaken to provide an enhanced opportunity for high grade A-level results. Some FE colleges have one-year residential courses. In a totally different context, foreign visits, expeditions and camps can all provide short-term residential experience while a particular programme is completed. Indeed, the DfES has indicated that it will be supporting a scheme under which all young people would at some stage go to camps as a short period of residential education. Thus residential time is seen officially as valuable in itself and also as providing a halfway house to independent living.

If there are clear objectives in mind, short-term residence can be highly beneficial. In Kahan (1994) the point is made that even a few days can allow a positive opportunity to contribute to a young person's overall well-being. Even in a short-term placement there may be benefits which may be summarised as follows:

- the feeling of enrichment from the residential experience in which there was a caring role;
- the acquisition of instrumental skills, such as using a telephone;
- the fact that issues which resulted in residence are addressed;
- the consensus among the staff, young people and parents about goals and how they should be achieved;
- the opportunity to work in small groups, to take responsibility and to have close relationships with staff.

Furthermore, if the period of residence is generally short, there is a rapid turnover of young people and the ethos of the establishment may be altered over a very limited time period. If the requirement is to change prevailing attitudes and the overall ambience, this can be achieved in, for example, sixth-form boarding schools, FE colleges, military training establishments and STCs in little over two years. In a boarding house which accommodates young people between the ages of 11 and 18, such a wholesale change is unlikely in under seven years.

In sharp contrast to short-term residence, very few young people may spend the best part of a lifetime in a residential institution. Some in special schools and health settings require permanent care beyond the scope of a family. In custodial care a few will have long-term incarceration but the most likely candidates for a lifetime are some of the occupants of forensic psychiatric units. Although, after the age of 18, they pass beyond the scope of residential education and care for young people, in certain cases, particularly in custodial care, the age of 18 appears to be an artificial dividing line. This is now recognised in the *Children (Leaving Care) Act* (2000), as a result of which local authorities may continue to have responsibility for certain young people until the completion of their education, when they may be well into their twenties.

In general the task, before they reach the age of 18, is to equip those young people who may never leave residence for a lifetime which will not involve independent living. For those in custodial care and possibly in forensic or other psychiatric units, personal and social development becomes a major issue. As far as possible, the young people need to develop resilience and inner strength together with lifelong interests. For young people with major health disabilities, the problems are different. For example, for extreme autism it may be a question of identifying appropriate environmental conditions which make them happy. Their appreciation of music, sounds or other sensations may be acute and the pleasure derived may equal or exceed the more sophisticated enjoyments of non-disabled young people. It may be possible to achieve much through art therapy.

Use of time

The passage of time alone, however it is used, may be beneficial. The young person will have matured and will have had time to reflect. The external environment may have changed and any problems which led to a period in residence may have disappeared. Clearly, if there is a programme which helps the young people develop and enhance their powers of reflection, the benefits are likely to be greater. As a result, it should be possible to define a minimal input from the establishment which will have a positive effect. The relationship between the possible transitions in the progress of the young people and time is summarised in Figure 5.3. Clearly if there is a relatively long stay, there is, potentially, time for integration so that at least some of the normal developmental transitions might take place before leaving. If the stay is short, there may be little time available between the completion of integration and the initiation of the leaving procedure. Indeed, in some cases, integration itself may not be realised before the young person has left the residence. Since the rite of passage into the establishment will vary according to the young person, it is obviously difficult to identify a minimum length of stay which can be in any way beneficial. Therefore, it is important that there is an attempt to have at least some input from the establishment which will help the young person in later life even during the period of integration.

In all settings there must be provision for education, normally based upon the National Curriculum. In addition, each sector has its own focus. All settings in the health sector have as their overriding concern medical problems, whether they be psychiatric, sensory impairment, physical disability, communication difficulty or other diseases and conditions. The young people are usually resident because treatment can only be provided effectively at the establishment or can, at least, be administered more effectively than at home. Some may have boarding needs as well as medical problems. For all, length of stay is governed by medical considerations.

In the custodial care sector, there are conflicting views about what the focus should be. Most would agree on containment and rehabilitation as a basic requirement but, beyond that there would probably be support for punishment. In itself, punishment offers little if anything in the way of a constructive

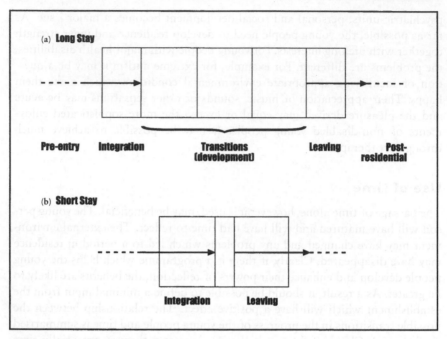

(a) **Long Stay**

Pre-entry   **Integration**   **Transitions**   **Leaving**   **Post-**
                                        (development)   **residential**

(b) **Short Stay**

Integration   **Leaving**

Figure 5.3   Time and development

programme. It is only rehabilitation which is positive and which allows meaningful comparison with programmes in the other sectors. In using the time
developmentally, the emphasis is upon behaviour. This involves confronting
offending behaviour and attempting to build survival skills for resisting re-
offending and establishing an independent life. Formal education is still vital,
particularly as many of the young people will have had at best a sketchy attendance record in school. Work on behaviour is closely related to concerns with
personal and social development and the length of time spent in residence is
governed not only by previous behaviour which resulted in the original
committal, but by current behaviour which can result in sentence length change.

Forensic psychiatry units are at the overlap of the medical and custodial sectors but, while they are custodial, they are governed by medical requirements.
At the overlap between the custodial and social sectors are secure units which,
in their approach, are more closely related to therapeutic communities and
other settings in the social sector. Containment is still crucial but the accent is
on a combination of behaviour and care. The length of time in residence may
be defined by a custodial order but normally there is some flexibility related to
the progress made by the young person.

The social sector as a whole, whether the young people are in special schools
for behaviour, emotional and social development difficulties or children's
homes, the accent is upon care. Antisocial behaviour is addressed, but in the

context of repairing or compensating for the damage the young people have suffered. In children's homes, the problems can be broadly defined as social but the categories of young people vary widely. In all the social settings, classroom education is fundamental although, as in the case of children's homes, the school may not be an integral part of the establishment. Children's homes are also distinguished by being generally much smaller units. Of all the settings, they are the nearest approach, in theory at least, to the family model. Length of stay is dictated ideally by the needs of the young people but, particularly in the case of children's homes, there may be other considerations such as the time required to make alternative arrangements including fostering, placement in a special boarding school or entry to a mainstream boarding school.

In all the sectors provision for formal education is basic, but in the education sector it is the focus. The programme is built around the curriculum and, since there is no other overriding concern as in the other three sectors, there is time for a greater range of activities in the extra-curricular field (Lambert *et al.*, 1970).

Given the time available it may be seen that FE colleges and boarding schools have an advantage over all the other sectors in developing residential or boarding education. However, in many ways this advantage remains more a question of potential. It has been only relatively recently, as society has changed and the boarding population has changed, that the need for a definite emphasis upon personal and social development has been taken seriously. There have always been boarding schools which adopted a holistic approach but these were comparatively rare. Perhaps one reason for the lack of focus has been the assumption that young people in boarding schools are 'normal' and will develop 'normally' among their peer group as, it was assumed, would be the case in their own families. It is now generally understood that while there may be steady progress by the majority, there will always be some young people with problems and it is the responsibility of the boarding school to address these problems.

Thus a consideration of the use of time in the context of the young people in residence provides some guidelines for practice, particularly in the realm of the transfer of expertise from one setting or sector to another. Thoughts about time also raise a number of interesting questions and problems to which there are no obvious answers. However, in an attempt to solve the problems, the thought and reflection undertaken by residential staff is likely to be of value in itself.

Time and staff

For staff, time begins with preparations following appointment. On arrival there should be a staff induction programme, in which the newcomer is introduced, in as much detail as possible, to the human and physical environments together with aspects of the external environment relevant to them. Above all there should be an emphasis on all the requirements for child protection, supervising and caring for groups of young people and combating likely crises and emergencies, such as fire. As an example of good practice in Australia, residential staff should have run a fire drill successfully before being allowed to take unsupervised charge of a group of young people. In boarding schools there is the particular issue of the induction of Gap assistants from abroad. As with the young people, there is a period of adjustment until new members of the residential staff are fully integrated into the staff team and the operation of the establishment. Thus, the transition time into the establishment can vary widely, depending upon a variety of factors from personal diligence to background knowledge and sympathy with the aims of the establishment.

Once settled, there may be a number of different roles expected. This is most obviously the case in boarding schools where many if not most of the residential staff are also members of the teaching staff. The main advantages of this arrangement are that most staff tend to gain their status with the young people by their performance as teachers. It is certainly difficult for non-teaching residential staff in such schools to reach equality of esteem. The argument that, as a teacher, the residential staff member sees the young people in a different light, is considerably less strong. If the individual is a subject specialist, it is unlikely that more than a limited number of boarders from the relevant house will be taught. If both teaching and pastoral care roles are undertaken, the result must be relatively stressful and extremely tiring. There is certainly an argument for specialist residential staff, a point accepted in many girls' boarding schools. The dual role of education and care can also lead to conflict over time in that there are likely to be problems concerning the differing demands and expectations of the boarding as opposed to the academic.

The dual role problem appears in modified form if at all in the other sectors. In FE colleges, some lecturers may be resident tutors but residences are normally run by designated residential staff. In special schools, there are likely to be specialist members of residential staff and teachers are likely to be involved more at a recognisably pastoral level. In the other sectors, there are rarely the equivalents to boarding school houses. In children's homes, numbers are generally so small that there are no formal sub-units. In custodial care, there are divisions of the young people by location but, other than in perhaps some competitive sense, they are hardly developed as separate entities. In the health sector, the young people may be separated according to need and the basic unit may be the ward or group of wards. An approximate summary of the situation would be that in boarding schools the house assumes greater importance than the school in the personal and social development of the young people. In all the other sectors the establishment predominates over any separate units (Figure 2.4). From the staff viewpoint one result of this fact may well be that integration with all the other residential staff is likely to be slower in boarding schools than in other types of setting, in all of which residential staff can work together while the young people are engaged in education. Conversely, integration with the young people in general may be quicker in boarding schools.

For residential staff in all sectors, the major distinction is between duty and non-duty time. The components of non-duty time will vary considerably according to whether the staff member is residential within the setting or lives away from it. This issue has generated considerable discussion which continues in various guises. Twenty to thirty years ago it would have been considered beneficial to have staff with families living on the campus. For all types of young people, this would have provided a demonstration of family life and should have rendered the environment more homely (Chapter 2). Apart from the ethos imparted, there are the obvious advantages of having more staff readily available for activities of all kinds and able to offer assistance in emergencies. Given the problems and costs of providing family accommodation, there has been a general move away from having residential staff in all types of setting except boarding schools. It is now increasingly common to have sleeping-in accommodation for duty staff. Sleeping-in staff may be more readily available and possibly potentially more effective than staff living with their families, particularly if they are housed in separate buildings. However, there must be losses in the lack of a family presence, particularly in those settings for which the model is the family. A further variation occurs in settings in which night-time problems, such as possible abuse of young people by their peers, are anticipated. Staff need to be particularly vigilant and are deployed as night-time patrols with the required number of staff always available.

The appreciation of the significance of time is fundamental to the developmental approach to young people, as discussed in Hunt and Sullivan (1974). The development of the young person is seen not as a series of self-sufficient incidents but as progress through a number of stages until fuller transition is apparent. To be used effectively, the model depends upon meticulous monitoring, assessment and record keeping by staff. These activities should occupy a significant part of the staff time spent in residential or boarding education and care.

On a personal level, time also presents opportunities for staff self-development, training and gaining new experience. Time spent observing and discussing practice with colleagues is vital if personal progress is to be made (Mallinson and Thomas, 1984). Time is also required for reading, reflection, keeping records and writing reports. Much of the time required for these various occupations will necessarily be taken from non-duty time. If the unselfish donation of time is to be encouraged, support for residential staff should be a core value for the establishment (McDerment, 1988).

At a more advanced staff level, time is a basic concern in all aspects of leadership (Hills and Child, 2000) and in the management of the main constituents of the operational residential setting: resources, environment and quality. Human resources constitute the most important concern of management (Investors in People UK, 2000). More time is likely to be beneficially spent in the recruitment and selection of staff, staff training and team development than on

any other issue (Payne, 2000). Physical resources each have their own time commitment ranging from consumables to the fabric and long-term wear and tear.
Since it is related to all types of resource, finance, whether in raising money or
balancing the budget or planning for the future, will be a major consumer of
time. The upkeep of the environment overlaps with physical resources and
includes not only the fabric and any grounds but all the service systems, the
maintenance of which is vital for the effective operation of the establishment.
At a more general level still, quality summarises all aspects of management. For
the parent, the inspector or the senior manager aspects of total quality will be
readily apparent. Time spent reviewing the complete operation of the setting in
the light of the philosophy, ethos, aims and objectives will not be wasted.
Another way of looking at time is that it is likely to be required for the different managerial elements in varying lengths. For example, for budget production
time periods are likely to be short and intense, while for quality control there
should be a continuous relatively limited expenditure of time. Looking further
ahead and more generally, time is of particular consequence in considering the
management of continuity and change.

Continuity implies the conservation and positive development of all that
seems effective and appropriate. If the setting is successfully fulfilling its aims
and the aims are sufficiently forward-looking, there must be hesitancy in intro-
ducing change, particularly radical change. If change is introduced as a result of
the demands of society then these demands themselves require at least some
discussion. Clearly if there is a significant mismatch between the aims of the
setting and the needs of society, change must be considered. Even more, if there
appear to be discrepancies between the aims and the needs of the young people,
something must be done. Indeed, the most appropriate overall balance to be
achieved is that between the aims of the establishment, which incorporate the
ideals from the past, and the changing needs of the young people who enter the
establishment.

Change need not be market-led but may come about as a result of innovation
and improved practice. In the custodial sector, change is being introduced as a
result of work in a number of special units associated with YOIs. In many children's homes a degree of specialisation has been introduced, which allows the
characteristics of the young people who might best be helped to be defined.
Such a procedure may become increasingly common in all sectors. Each setting
is unique and needs to identify its particular strengths. If such strengths and
specialisms were identified throughout residential and boarding education and
care, this would allow matching between the young people and their requirements, a procedure which in all settings except those for which there are very
clear definitions of needs, has a tendency to range from the superficial to the
haphazard.

Whatever the reason for change care must be taken, as far as possible, to
ensure that neither the scale nor the rate is in excess of what the establishment can absorb, while retaining a basic continuity. Many boarding schools

and establishments in the health and social sectors have shown great resilience in the face of change but major and rapid change has certainly resulted in the demise of some. The custodial sector, having seen more fundamental changes than any other, has, in its present form, had relatively little experience of continuity. In the best-balanced settings, much change will occur inadvertently and incrementally as a result of a proactive approach to good practice.

Daily living

To examine time specifically in a particular setting it seems appropriate to select the smallest reasonable measure, the day, and the longest, the entire career of a young person in association with the establishment. Clearly the activities of the day will vary depending upon the stage of the week, the time of year and most particularly upon the characteristics and categories of the young people. There will be even greater variation around the career as a measurement since length of stay, stages and transitions are likely to differ widely according to the young people involved, their personal and social developmental starting point and type of setting.

Daily living allows formative evaluation and, if necessary, the amendment of procedures, whereas a consideration of the full career can only provide, for the individual, summative evaluation. Both, in differing ways, can allow an assessment to be made of the characteristics and effectiveness of the setting. A detailed welfare audit of events over two or three days should provide sufficient evidence to identify concerns. If the investigation is to find indicators which may be used to characterise the ethos of the particular setting and place it accurately on the family-to-formal continuum, then experience of daily living by the investigator is vital. Such action research provides the basis for good, evidence-based practice. The total performance of a number of young people at the end of their careers provides some evaluation of the overall effectiveness of the setting.

Daily living represents the modal position within the setting (Berry, 1975). It is what normally occurs and therefore excludes weekends, if they differ from weekdays, and special days. The concept of the modal day allows a distinction to be made between the staff who are part of the human environment and those who may work at times within the establishment but are essentially the external environment.

The basic requirement is that the philosophy, aims, values, principles or what is encapsulated by the Mission Statement are expressed in policies, procedures and practice to meet the needs of the particular group of young people (Sinclair and Gibbs, 1998). As there are likely to be variations in those needs, a second key consideration is that time is allowed for work with individuals. It is the young people who are central to the day. It must be remembered that, other than in perhaps a fairly superficial way, many of the young people have not chosen to

be in the establishment whereas for the staff there has been a conscious decision. Not all the young people could be categorised as involuntary clients but
the subject is clearly a consideration throughout residential and boarding education and care (Trotter, 1999). Some boarders and a few in special boarding
schools and some health settings, together with probably the majority of residents in FE colleges and military training establishments, may be thought to
have made a conscious decision that involved residential living. Other young
people had boarding need and some had specific health or care needs or were
referred to residence.

Apart from free time, the day may be divided into formal education and/or
treatment and residential education. In all the settings there is an element of
classroom education even though it may not actually take place in a classroom.
The classroom may not be within the establishment and, for some settings, most
notably children's homes, departure for school and arrival from school are key
events. All sectors will require liaison between the residential staff and the
teachers.

For the young person leaving the establishment for school, the accent is on
smoothing the passage from one community to another and ensuring that the
young people are not characterised or particularly stigmatised as from the children's home or some other similar setting. With in-house education, a focus is
upon enhancing the difference between the classroom and the living unit. In a
boarding school, the house may have many characteristics in common with the
school including a library and a room used as a classroom, but it is essentially
'home'. The approach of the residential staff member in the classroom is likely
to be quite different from that adopted in the boarding house. This is a potential role conflict which appears to be relatively easily overcome in most schools.
In boarding schools in which the teaching and residential staff are quite separate, the effect is somewhere between that of an external and an internal school.

For sectors other than educational, a further set part of the day is likely to
concern health and medical practice, behaviour issues or focused care concerns.
These may require the daily attendance of highly specialised staff who then
constitute part of the human environment. Medical specialists, psychologists,
psychiatrists, therapists and social workers who are not members of the educational or the residential staff provide an element little represented in boarding
schools except on an occasional peripatetic basis. However, in the larger boarding schools there will be full-time nurses attached to the school medical centre
and in most boarding schools there will be matrons who have received some
medical training.

Residential and boarding education

The other major component of the daily timetable, which overlaps behavioural
issues and even more markedly care concerns, is residential or boarding education which results from living and learning together. This may be expressed as

a shared commitment to the goal of learning from the experience of living and/or working together (Charterhouse, 2001).

Potential support for learning in the residential environment may be offered by all staff, but in particular by the residential staff together with the peer group. The external network of specialists and non-specialists can play a role but the burden must fall on the permanent members of staff.

In business school terms, the approach of staff may be categorised as predominantly any of the following: task-, process- or people-orientated. The multi-faceted nature of residential work means that, in all sectors, all three need to be strongly in evidence. The daily routine needs to be completed for the benefit of the community and this comprises essentially a series of tasks. Policies must be implemented by set procedures especially in connection with events such as abuse, bullying or the receipt of complaints, and these are clearly processes. However, the focus is on the young people and, important as the other two criteria are, people orientation must be the most crucial if residential education is to develop and flourish. For living and learning, the staff should not only provide security in all senses for the young people but should use the total environment as a teaching aid and should provide an example through their own lives.

The total role is similar to parenting but residential staff are not surrogate parents. However, they may have been delegated parental responsibility and they should act like reasonable parents. As appropriate, the staff share the routines with the young people, particularly the communal activities such as mealtimes. In all sectors, there will be young people who have never sat down at a table for a meal in a formal fashion with adults who talk to each other and to them. While eating together is in many ways the foremost of all communal functions in a family, as a result of the hectic pace of life, the dislocation of families and the influence of television, for some families it has become almost non-existent. Sitting around the fire in a group, as a family, listening to music or watching television are further occasions when living and learning can take place.

The staff come equipped with their life experiences, their interests, hobbies, skills, knowledge and enthusiasms. For a young person, any one of these might spark an interest that could last a lifetime. It is also worth making the point that there may also be certain staff characteristics, particularly attitudes, which are best not transferred to the young people. Small events – successes, misdemeanors, breakages, manners, courtesy and many others – may be used to teach or reinforce lessons for life (Clough, 2000).

In particular, the young people can be encouraged to put themselves in somebody else's place. An apparently minor event such as a comment may appear small to the person who makes it but it may be a very serious issue for the person to whom it is directed. To hide someone's glasses may seem just a joke but to the person with very short sight it can be extremely demeaning. While it cannot be expected that all the young people in a group will like each other, at least they can be brought to a state where they have some understanding of each other's needs.

In all sectors, the potential for peer group learning is being given greater prominence. To an extent formally, but in fact largely informally, the peer group has always been a major source of residential education in boarding schools. This has resulted from the way in which boarding has developed and the high ratios of young people to staff. An implication is that the peer group is relatively benign, but worries on this score have tended to limit association in the custodial sector. However, for all young people in residence, the success of subsequent independent living depends, in no small measure, upon the ability to live with the peer group.

As part of the living and learning, the staff, of course, also learn from the young people. They increase their knowledge of each individual and thereby enhance their own practice. Furthermore, they may learn or improve their skills. With the increasing dominance of the electronic age, there has been something of a role reversal in teaching. Young people, having been brought up with computers, video games and other such devices, have normally developed far greater facility than people of older generations. This situation clearly presents opportunities for developing the self-esteem of the young people and also retaining their concentration for relatively lengthy periods. Indeed, under the appropriate circumstances, video games may be used as an effective substitute for role-play exercises.

The environment itself may also play a significant part in living and learning. The human environment comprises more than its individual component parts in that the ethos, culture and expectations should all be apparent to the sensitive observer. The 'therapeutic' orientation of the community exercises a strong influence upon the young people and their behaviour (Lennox, 1982). The physical environment may also be important in that it can provide an obvious demonstration of the values of the establishment. What is the division between public and private rooms? Do the staff take their meals at a separate table? From which areas are the young people excluded and for what reasons? In what ways in its layout does it approach a family home? On a scale from authoritarian to participative, where would the setting be rated? There are many other factors involved with the physical environment including in particular personal space, furnishings, services and decor. Are the young people consulted on how rooms are decorated? How private is personal space?

In most settings the young people have some role to play in the operation and maintenance of the establishment. Practical life-skill competence, a prerequisite for independence, is an important aspect of the living and learning environment.

Routines provide the framework of the normal day and, in their regularity and consistency, offer support for the young people (Berry, 1975). Many young people entering all settings, and most going into some, will not have experienced the discipline of such a programme and will not have realised the importance of adhering closely to a timetable. In group living, it is only by completing each event on time that the full programme can run. One person's negligence, even over some seemingly insignificant happening, can negatively affect the rest of the group or even the community. Predictability and dependability provide reassurance for the young people and allow the synchronisation of their 'rhythms' with those of the staff and environment (Maier, 1987). This idea ties in closely with the responsibilities of good parenting (Coles, 2000).

Apart from fixed times such as waking, bedtime and mealtimes, there are various routines, chores and possibly even traditions. Traditions tend to be associated with boarding schools but, in various forms and with modifications, some have appeared in almost all settings. For example, there may not be a purpose-built chapel but there is likely to be a quiet room for reflection and spiritual welfare. Furthermore, although the UK may be described in some quarters as post-Christian, members of other religions may well retain their fervour and wish to practise their religion in a thoughtful way.

One routine, common in much of residential living, is the roll-call which is, for different reasons, crucial in all settings. In custodial care the point is obvious, but in homes and schools it is vital for their own safety to know the whereabouts of all the young people. A careless approach to taking the roll-call by one member of staff can lead to major problems. It is an interesting exercise to calculate, during any week, the longest period of time the absence of a young person might remain undetected. Another routine is cleaning, and in most settings there is a certain responsibility for the tidiness of personal space and possibly parts of the public space. As in families domestic duties are shared increasingly between husband and wife, training in domesticity for both girls and boys develops important life skills.

The framework of routines subsumes the organisational component of daily living. However, the major part of daily living, outside formal education or specialised treatment, is likely to be occupied by the programme of activities. Whether these are formal or informal, individual or group, they all require a degree of preparation and certainly a preview. Some will be purely for leisure and others will be orientated towards an intentional learning bias although any can provide effective living and learning opportunities. An example is team games which offer a number of opportunities ranging from team-work and acceptance of decisions to leadership and helping the less gifted. A great deal may be learned about the young people by watching their performance and attitude during a game of football. Are they team players? Do they accept valid decisions? Can they give and take instructions? What are their reactions to winning and losing?

The focus of the activities may be upon a specific learning aim or a particular individual or group of young people (Doel and Sawdon, 1999). For example, a pastime may be introduced to allow an isolate to be drawn into a group or to offer an opportunity for responsibility to an individual. The sharing of a common hobby between a member of staff and a young person allows just the kind of learning situation which occurs in a family. The mutual interest develops a loyalty in the relationship which allows the staff member to offer guidance, on a variety of issues, more effectively to the young person.

During daily living, there are also likely to be unintended outcomes and incidents. A review of the day's events will reveal beneficial outcomes which may be used to improve practice. Incidents may clearly be good and should be appropriately rewarded, but may concern breakages, acting out, conflict and displays of antisocial behaviour which must be addressed and recorded in the incident book.

Whether it is in relatively exotic pursuits such as mountaineering or scuba diving, in mundane activities such as riding a bicycle on the main road or tackling in football, or in personal everyday issues such as making one's opinion known, all involve some level of risk. If there is no course of action which is clear-cut, the probabilities are weighed mentally and a decision is made. Whatever that decision there will be some risk, but under normal circumstances the intention is to take the course with a lower or probably the least risk attached. Since normal life is about decisions and risks, if young people in residential and boarding education and care are to survive successfully in life after their period of residence, they need to be exposed to risk (Chapter 2).

The role of staff is to calculate what is an acceptable risk. In implementing an activity, the staff member is also taking a risk. Therefore, it is wise to keep a detailed record. As far as possible, it is appropriate for the young people to be involved in such risk assessment as they will need to carry out such a decision-making process for themselves in later life. The risk assessment procedure, modified appropriately, needs to be carried out to assess and address potential hazards in both the physical and the human environment. It may also be used, in a very specific form, to check on compliance with the framework components. Essentially, the process involves the identification of actual or potential hazards, a forecast of the possible risk for the young people and staff which can be attached to each and action to minimise satisfactorily or eliminate the problem. For a faulty electrical fitting, this would involve its rapid replacement. For a visit outside the establishment, considerations would include transport, the mix of young people making the visit, the staff requirements and any specific problems which might arise at the venue. Risk assessment grades into the preview which all residential staff should conduct before a period of duty.

When intervening (Chapter 2) on behalf of a particular young person, it will be realised that there may be some follow-up action when the staff member is not present. When should young people be protected and when should they be left to fight their own battles? The experienced practitioner will be aware that, in a particular situation, a threshold has been crossed and there is likely to be an incident. When does friendly banter become bullying? It is clear what is happening but intervention may, in the longer term, make the situation worse. This is a case in which the threshold of the young person being bullied and the member of staff, who is conversant with the bullying, may differ. In the end, the ultimate judge of whether bullying has occurred must be the person being bullied and, with experience and detailed knowledge of the young people, staff should be able to judge when a personal threshold has been crossed.

Daily living is the building block of residential life (Rose, 2002). Incremental changes are noted from day to day and allow the full picture of development to be obtained. However, effective developmental profiles can only be produced if staff are diligent in monitoring. The most minor events may merit thought and reflection, and seemingly trivial pieces of information may be significant in identifying the progress of an individual. In supervising the day, the overall aim is to achieve balance between all the conflicting pressures and forces so that risks are acceptable, and intervention is appropriate while living and learning is successfully achieved.

Transitions

The aggregation of monitored daily events produces a profile of development in which certain stages may be discerned. The stages may be considered thresholds in that they indicate distinct changes in behaviour (Hunt and Sullivan, 1974). They may be sharp but generally they will be relatively gradual and possibly characterised by a short period of atypical behaviour. Compared with the relative stability on either side, they represent change over a compressed period of time. To these stages within the establishment may be added those which precede and those which follow residence but which are in a tangible way connected to residence. The pre-residential stage would be concerned with preparations for arriving. In some sectors, notably health and custodial, this may be very short indeed and there may be almost no time for preparatory thought. The relevant period following residence would be one in which a definite link with the establishment had been retained. For some settings in the health sector there may be a medical need to retain close contact. For the educational sector, predominantly boarding schools, there is usually a definite attempt to retain a network of former pupils. In the social, custodial and some of the health settings, departure may be precipitate although the importance of some form of after-care is well recognised. The entire span from pre-entry to after-care may be seen as a set of transitions.

Monitoring and recording changes over varying time scales requires subtlety, thought and trained observational skills. It also needs diligence and tenacity to sit down and make notes at the end of a period of duty. In many establishments the situation is being eased by the user-friendly computer programs which allow all the significant details to be recorded in a few minutes. The analysis and interpretation of data to produce valid and reliable normative or summative assessment requires specialist knowledge and training and, for any establishment, is probably best set up initially with help from external experts. Once the system has been set up, maintenance and adjustment to a changing environment may be managed internally.

One advantage which residential settings have over non-residential establishments is that they can, with some validity, claim a reasonable part of the credit for the progress made by the young people. Advances may have been made entirely as a result of maturation but, if many of the young people make definite progress, then it is reasonable to suppose that the establishment has some responsibility. Thus there seems to be an interesting balance in that, the more a particular setting approaches a total institution (Lambert, 1975), the more results may be directly attributed to its programme. However, the problems of total institutions have been well aired and there is concern in all sectors for openness and as close a relationship as possible with the external environment. The boarding schools are now very much more open institutions than they were in the early 1970s during Lambert's surveys. As a result, it is reasonable to conclude that the credit for success in boarding schools must be shared with parents and others in the external environment. In children's homes, responsibility for progress depends upon both the home and the school. In custodial and many social and health care settings, relations with the external environment are limited and success over the period of residence must be largely attributable to the establishment.

Changes and thresholds in the developmental components have already been discussed (Chapter 4) and, in the context of transitions, it is the overall rather than the individual developmental changes which are of significance. Broadly speaking, the changes occur with age and enhanced conceptual level. However, each young person is different and the mix of components which allows judgement as to when a particular stage has been reached will vary. If the three stages are accepted at face value, they help define the most suitable environment at that stage. In general terms, the matching environment would be, for the unsocialised stage, highly structured and relatively tightly managed and, for the independent stage, unstructured with guidance and an accent on autonomy. The point is that development and the behaviours by which it is detected are a function of the individual and the environment. This is recognised in all settings but distinctions may be seen. For example, in FE colleges, military training establishments, children's homes, therapeutic communities and boarding schools the focus is considerably more upon the person than upon the environment, whereas in custodial and many health care settings the environment predominates. Within that approximation there will be many variations but it is instructive to consider the balance between the two in any particular setting.

Pre-arrival

Pre-arrival time, if available, is important to allow preparations for what, in most cases, would be a significant life change (Brearley et al., 1980). Even for young people who have experienced residence away from home, entry into a new establishment, with the necessity of adjusting to all the facets of life, is bound to be somewhat forbidding. If adequate preparations, including preliminary visits, can be made, at least some mental adjustment can have taken place. In the educational sector, it is expected that there will be visits of parents and young people before entry, although this is not, of course, possible in the majority of cases with foreign young people. In the health sector, other than in cases of emergency, there is also likely to be some reasonable prior warning before arrival. For a variety of reasons, in the social and custodial sectors there may be no time for mental or physical preparation at all. Young people frequently come to children's homes as a result of some action beyond their control, such as family breakdown. Therefore nobody could have made any preparations and the situation is exacerbated by the very limited number of residential places available at any one location. There may be some warning for young people entering residence as a result of behavioural, emotional and social development difficulties but in many cases it will be very limited. For the remainder, the decision for referral tends to be followed by the action. Furthermore, since the number of beds is likely to be very limited, the exact location of the setting is determined more by the availability of accommodation than proximity to home location. This problem is being addressed as far as possible but some settings have such low total capacities that placement is unlikely to be fully appropriate.

Ideally, matching would involve the young person and a specific establishment but, for much of residential care, the best hope is that the young person at least ends up in the appropriate sector. There are young people with very similar characteristics who are in the educational, health, social and custodial sectors. When more appropriate indicators for settings have been developed, it is hoped that this issue can be more effectively addressed. Of all the settings, only the boarding schools have a sufficiently large number of places and establishments, nationally spread, for matching to be a current realistic possibility.

Induction

The major transition is from a non-residential situation into residential and boarding education and care. For most young people, this means leaving home and familiar surroundings and substituting for them what must seem a significantly more impersonal environment. Clearly there are considerable variations in all stages of this procedure. The home may be a loving, supportive environment or it may be totally dysfunctional, or it may be merely a resting place among unfamiliar people. The residential environment may vary considerably in size from a children's home of six or fewer to an FE college or boarding school of several hundred. Even if the reception unit is only sixty or fewer, variation by a factor of ten makes a vast difference to all aspects of arrival. In special schools, numbers will be considerably less and in health sector and social settings less again. In custodial care, there is a distinction between YOIs, which normally number hundreds, and STCs, which average around forty young people.

Reception will also vary substantially according to whether the transition is characterised as selection or referral. Selection can, of course, imply a two-way procedure. The establishment may have been selected by the parent, with or without the help of the young person, or the setting may have selected the young person. In cases in which there are limited numbers of places, selection is supply-led and this situation obtains in many health, education and social settings. Boarding schools are rather different on account of the relatively large number of places available. Demand clearly varies according to the perceived quality of the school, particularly if it has a noted specialisation. For example, competition is effectively worldwide for those schools specialising in music. The custodial sector together with some health and social settings are subject to referrals. Any possible selection is likely to be carried out by the authorities although there should be consultation with those who have parental responsibility.

Geographically, between the home and the setting, there may be, as a result of the selection or the referral procedure, a long distance. The young person arrives in wholly unfamiliar surroundings knowing that visits and home contact are going to be particularly difficult. This problem can occur in any of the sectors although in boarding schools there is an increasing tendency for most of the young people to come from the local region. The main exception in boarding schools is the foreign element which may reach 30 per cent or more of the boarding population, and introduces a further range of specific issues. The problem of dealing with young people from different ethnic and cultural backgrounds is likely to be shared by all the types of setting but the number of young people coming directly from abroad is likely to be very limited. Only in boarding schools, FE colleges, military establishments and particularly homes for refugee children are numbers likely to be significant. Issues of race, religion, the procurement of the appropriate documentation concerning their academic and medical background and their level of adjustment are set out in Holgate (2001). Problems of transition into the establishment will be more acute than those of most indigenous young people, depending upon the degree of prior preparation. When such young people join the establishment, they may require some positive discrimination, although care must be taken that this does not raise too many problems with their peers.

For any of the young people, there should be a formal induction procedure so that, before the onset of education and possibly treatment, the physical environment, the peer group and the basic procedures have been introduced. However, the major factor upon entry into residence is the 'acclimatisation' which is required. There will be an initial period when there appears to be no substitute at all for home and life is at best transitory. During this time, attempts will be made at familiarisation and behaviour is likely to be, in many respects, atypical. Once there has been sufficient acclimatisation for a personal balance to be reached, the young person can be integrated into the establishment. For some young people this passage is relatively rapid, while for a few it may never be achieved. Clearly the possibility of completing the rite of passage is linked closely to the length of stay in the establishment. Another influential factor is the degree of control exercised by the staff. In general, it appears that a young person becomes integrated more rapidly into a formal, more disciplined establishment rather than one in which a *laissez-faire* approach governs. However, this does raise the question of what integration actually means and how it is perceived by residential peers and staff.

For some young people, particularly during the transition stage of entry into the establishment, motivation to run away is at its strongest. Apart from previous experience of absconding, among the factors causing such motivation are:

- negative feelings about the establishment;
- homesickness;
- treatment or perceived treatment by staff;
- peer group pressure;
- bullying, discrimination or abuse.

(Wade and Biehal, 1998)

The subject is of relevance throughout residential and boarding education and care and staff should be aware of the establishment's procedures. Any investigation needs to include the peer group, young people in the same group, public rooms, living accommodation, the sick bay, any grounds and any sports facilities together with records of external visits and appointments. After a thorough search, a report is made immediately to the member of staff with responsibility for emergencies. Liaison may then be made with those who have parental responsibility, the police and other necessary professionals.

Leaving

On leaving the establishment, wherever the final destination, another major transition occurs. In all settings, care is taken to prepare young people for leaving (Burgess, 1981). Ideally they should not only want to go but they should feel that the full range of benefits have been received and a stage of life has been completed. For some, the key event will be reintegration into their families (Bullock *et al.*, 1998b), for others initiation into the world of work, further study or the search for a sustainable lifestyle. In the health care settings, the appropriate time for leaving is allied to medical decisions. In the custodial and much of the social sector, benefits are probably only appreciated later and there could have been a desire to leave from the moment of entry. In FE colleges and boarding schools, if the residential education has been effective, there should be some coincidence between the feeling of the young people on the right time for leaving and the actual date of departure. Of all the sectors, the educational sector is the one in which leaving is generally and most obviously planned and positive. For many settings in the other sectors, the future is largely unknown and the young person has, often virtually instantaneously, to resort to basic life skills.

These issues raise the important question of the proximate and the ultimate aims of residence. Are the aims predominantly or wholly to fit the young people for life immediately after leaving the setting or are they aimed at the longer expanse of life? In all sectors there is undoubtedly the hope that what has been learned will provide a support well into the future but it is extremely difficult, if not impossible, to evaluate long-term success with any validity. National Minimum Standards all address the short term and none take into account the longer term effects of residence. For some types of setting the internal focus represents an improvement. For example, the custodial sector always tends to be judged on rates of recidivism. Young people may have received first-class residential education within the establishment but, on leaving and entering the environment over which the establishment has no control, they re-offend. All that may be said with any certainty is that the establishment was unable to provide them with sufficient resilience to resist the effects of perhaps their families, their peers or other elements of the environment in which they had previously offended. In some cases, halfway houses and a change of location have resulted in the lowering of re-offending rates. The health sector is chiefly concerned with medical success and this is largely achieved within the establishments. Such success may be in the form of a cure or in the inculcation of the skills required for independence and normal living. The social sector, in general terms, tries to prepare the young people for a self-supporting life. As with the custodial sector, if such young people are convicted of crimes or found guilty of antisocial behaviour, the establishment tends to be blamed. Boarding schools, like the health sector, have always been judged primarily upon their internally generated results. If the young people offend in a significant way, the boarding school may be mentioned by the media but it is not normally specifically held responsible.

The aims of the settings themselves may be divided into a focus on the internal or very short term after leaving and an emphasis upon the more general hopes for the future. As far as possible within the time constraints, preparations are made for both short-term and long-term aims. However, under normal circumstances, the more time that has elapsed since leaving, the less the individual setting may be expected to accept responsibility for what happens. Perhaps the boarding schools can be distinguished in that their long-term aims are often very general and couched in terms of a happy, fulfilled, useful and successful life. For the health, custodial and care sectors respectively, the basic aims are a healthy and medically fit life, a life free from further offences and an independent normal life.

For most young people leaving residential and boarding education and care, there is likely to be at least an increased degree of independence, and preparations for this may be seen as covering three broad aspects:

1   Enabling young people to build and maintain relationships with others.
2   Enabling young people to develop their self-esteem.
3   Teaching practical and financial skills and knowledge.

(DoH, 1999)

A list of skills and knowledge for which many young people are inadequately prepared is provided in the same volume and includes the following:

- how to shop for, prepare and cook food;
- eating a balanced diet;
- laundry, sewing and mending and other housekeeping skills;
- how to carry out basic household jobs;
- safety in the home and first aid;
- the cost of living;
- household budgeting;
- health education;
- sexual education;
- applying for, and being interviewed for, a job;
- applying for a course of educational training;
- applying for social security benefits;
- applying for housing;
- registering for doctor and dentist;
- how to write a letter of complaint or to obtain advice.

After-care

After-care or continuing support, in which there is increasing interest, has different implications according to the sector of residence. However, all young people leaving residential and boarding education and care would benefit from advice and information together with a continued interest in their welfare. In particular, assistance may be needed for education and training or accommodation (DoH, 1991a). In the educational sector, the perception has always been that a particular stage of education was complete once the young person left. However, for a variety of reasons most schools and colleges have old pupils' associations and, through them, supportive programmes have been developed. Most of the young people concerned are likely to be relatively successful and therefore specific support is focused upon professional help. The other main concerns are predominantly social and nostalgic.

In the health sector, continuing medical support may be required and this constitutes the main form of after-care. For example, young people with sensory and/or physical difficulties may wish to keep in touch with developments in their particular field of disability. If no such help is needed, then contact may be severed, although some young people may continue with an interest in the activities of their former health and medical establishment, particularly in the case of the special schools. For the custodial sector, leaving has traditionally meant severance of ties. It is now realised that this is the sector which needs after-care most of all. If the young people are to be reintegrated into society and to live independently, they require a support network. Similarly, in the social sector, success for many young people must depend upon a measure of after-care. The young people from the social and custodial sectors are the most vulnerable but have the least developed support network. It is ironic that the former pupils of FE colleges and boarding schools, in the context of the residential and boarding sector by far the most likely to succeed in life, tend to receive the most after-care.

However, the picture is changing as it is increasingly revealed that much of the work in the custodial and social sectors can be nullified unless efforts are made to help settle the young people into society. There is now a wide variety of schemes, some run by local authorities and some by central government, which exist to help young people realise their potential and achieve successful independent living. For some young people, after-care at the age of 18 is particularly problematic since they continue to live in some form of institution. In the medical sector, some young people require such a high level of attention that they will always live in a health setting. For much the same reason some will remain in psychiatric settings, while for some young people, life will continue in a custodial setting. Of those who leave STCs at 15 years of age, some proceed to a YOI. For some, residence will be continuous in a YOI and then in an adult prison from age 16 to beyond age 18. In the social sector, some young people will leave and move into hostel accommodation. Now, with the *Children (Leaving Care) Act* (2000), local authorities have a continuing responsibility for young people who have been in their care and therefore it must be expected that conditions will improve. For the custodial settings, considerations of after-care are still largely in the experimental and pilot project stage.

This discussion calls into question the continuing use of the eighteenth birthday as a threshold. Some young people are mature at that age, others are still developing and the extension of local authority responsibility provides some recognition of this point. It is an interesting question as to what responsibility establishments have for the young people after they have left and to what age that responsibility continues. The boarding school sector has always envisaged a continuum from the school into life as the young people become part of the establishment's extended family. This positive concept in some modified form needs to be examined in the light of the other sectors (Kahan, 1994).

Average figures mean relatively little but may give an approximate overall picture. By the time they leave, some young people will have spent most of their lives in certain specialised health settings and possibly social care establishments, although this will almost certainly have included periods of fostering. In very broad terms, young people in secondary boarding schools will have spent 40 per cent of their lives attached to the establishment and, if they attended preparatory boarding schools first, this figure may rise to about 60 per cent. In custodial care, the percentage varies from about 10 per cent to 30 per cent. In the health sector in general, most are likely to have spent under 1 per cent but some as much as 40 per cent. Figures vary for the social settings but it would not be unusual for young people to have spent 35 per cent of their lives in a residential setting. These are mostly significant amounts of time and, given the high inputs of resources into all sectors, it is reasonable to expect that some guidance and support would remain available to the young people after the age of 18.

Chapter 6

The model and its applications

Using evidence from the varied types of setting in the four sectors which comprise the field, the fundamentals of the system which may be classified as residential and boarding education and care have been identified. This system has been analysed and the key components assembled into a model which has been developed and tested in the field and examined in detail in this book using examples from all the sectors. As each of the components has been discussed, it has been possible to relate it not only to its constitute parts but also to the other main components. Each component has offered a different viewpoint upon what must be the core of any residential or boarding establishment, the living and learning environment, and this has allowed cross-referencing of the various issues raised. The discussions have been illustrated by examples from all the different types of setting, thereby highlighting commonalities and differences, and suggesting potential for transfer. Examples of good practice in one type of setting may be considered for the possible benefit of the other sectors.

The model provides a coherent overview and, despite being used by government departments and at many meetings and conferences, has remained robust and resilient over the past three years. It appears parsimonious at the component level in that each is clear and distinctive and there is no replication. More significantly, no omissions have been suggested and in fact the model fits with other models of parts of the residential system (e.g. DoH, 2000a, 2000b). Furthermore, the model fulfils one key requirement in that it not only accounts for the issues raised but it also suggests further concepts and ideas not previously considered. Most important, it fits all the different types of settings and indicates clearly the possibilities of the transfer of good practice between them.

The application of the model in providing a summary of the system, any component of which may be developed further, has demonstrated a key aspect of its use. In an examination of a residential or boarding education and care setting, the model provides the basic plan which allows key issues, both negative and positive, to be pinpointed. Moreover, there are more specialised uses and there is potential to extrapolate from the model.

Training

Since the model summarises the residential and boarding education and care system, a major application is in the identification of staff training requirements. Furthermore, the location of training elements already completed may be seen within the perspective of the whole system. Indeed, the first iteration of the model was constructed during the early design phase of the Joseph Rowntree Foundation-funded course for staff training. At the start, acknowledged front-line practitioners were asked to set out their ideas on the material required. The various suggestions were grouped into potential modules and shown to practitioners representing all the main types of setting in the expectation that there would be significant variations in needs, at least by sector, if not by type of setting. In fact, there was a high degree of agreement that all the potential modules should be included. To take two examples, whether violent and threatening behaviour is likely to occur in a particular establishment at most once a year or on a daily basis, staff still need to know how to deal with it. Support by residential staff for educational studies is seen to be vital across all sectors. As a result, it was decided that, rather than a series of separate courses, one for each sector, there could and should be one generic course covering the requirements at certificate, diploma and degree level. The agreed material was then checked against all current NVQs and related courses and all service Standards. This process was facilitated by the fact that, while the course was being designed, the author was a member of four Training Organisation for the Personal Social Services (TOPSS) committees which were producing National Minimum Standards. The material which emerged from these various procedures to cover training requirements was then divided into modules which were checked extensively by email, using a review body of about fifty experts and a series of eight regional meetings.

With general agreement on the material, it was decided that the key level would be that of the diploma in that the degree level and the certificate level, respectively above and below the diploma level, could be derived from it. In addition, the diploma is significant not only as a Year 2 university course but also as a post-qualifying diploma for those who already have degree-level qualifications. Frameworks were then constructed to cover the modules for the generic diploma-level course and it was from these that the model was developed. Subsequently, the model served as the basis for the development and trialling of the course at diploma level together with the production of the certificate and degree level courses.

While the model indicates the common training elements at each level, the weightings accorded to each vary somewhat depending upon the sector. For example, while all four are concerned with it, the physical environment is of particular relevance in the health and custodial sectors. Given the nature of most treatments, the idea of transitions is of least relevance in the health sector (Figure 6.1). Besides the weightings, there are certain elements which are unique to specific sectors,

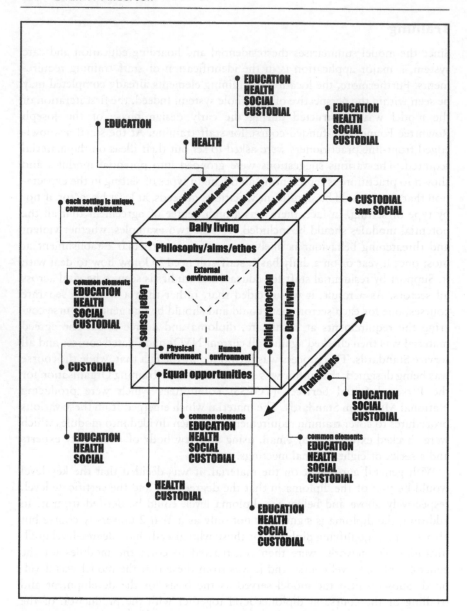

Figure 6.1　Model for training

including, for example, specialised medical techniques in the health sector and search techniques in the custodial sector. These are further developments beyond the scope of the model as described and they are grouped, for each sector, in a separate module. They are derived from the model in that, for example, considerations of security are important in all types of setting but added precautions need to be taken in custodial care. Health and medical elements are important as part of developmental monitoring in all sectors but clearly there are particular needs in settings which care for young people with sensory and/or physical difficulties.

The model has been used not only for course design and development but also for the production of material for training days. In that context, it allows those attending the day to see not only how the particular elements under discussion fit into the overall pattern of residential and boarding education and care but also how they relate to other elements. For example, the philosophy/ aims/ethos element of the framework components provides the starting point for a programme to monitor the personal and social development of the young people. Considerations of child protection include not only the prevention of abuse and discrimination but also the provision of a healthy lifestyle and an environment in which the young people can develop towards their full potential.

For training purposes, the environmental components demonstrate how the system operates on a daily basis and allows the staff training required to address the needs of the young people to be identified. The relationships between the three environments highlight aspects such as security, emergency planning and relationships with parents and those with parental responsibility. The framework components together comprise the safeguards for the welfare of the young people and provide a synopsis of all the key legal requisites for staff. The individuality of each setting is illustrated by its philosophy which should be used by staff to generate the aims and objectives for the developmental components.

The developmental components illustrate the use of daily activities to monitor the progress of the young people so that remedial action may be taken if necessary and the momentum of the establishment towards the achievement of its objectives may be monitored. For the very short term and the long term, the time components provide a synopsis of all the activities within the system from a completely different viewpoint. A consideration of transitions extends the coverage of the model appropriately beyond the setting from pre-entry to after-care.

Management

As agreed by the TOPSS National Steering Group during the preparation of the National Occupational Standards for Managers in Residential Child Care, management has to be allied to good practice (Horwath and Morrison, 1999). A manager should not be seen as superior to a top-quality practitioner and all managers should be effective practitioners (Burton, 1998; Clough, 2000). Since the model provides a plan of the system and how it operates, it offers a framework for management in residential and boarding education and care.

Within the system, there are managerial roles at various levels from junior to senior. At one level there is the newly qualified staff member, managing a small group of young people, and at the other the overall principal, head or manager of the school, home or specialised setting. With regard to the human environment, the former may be working on conflict resolution with two young people or trying to introduce an isolate to a group while the latter is managing the full daily programme of activities (Reynolds *et al.*, 2003). In either case, the model, as set out in detail, indicates the managerial commitment to each element. Put another way, at certificate level there needs to be an awareness particularly of child protection, what to do in emergencies and the philosophy of the establishment. With this background, the staff member can manage a section of the human environment, given some knowledge of the physical and external environments, and can contribute effectively to emergency and crisis intervention. At the diploma level, the staff member is likely to be involved in self-management (Megginson *et al.*, 1996) and team management (Brown and Bourne, 1999; Coulshed and Mullender, 2001; Hawkins and Shohet, 2000). As director, principal or head, the role is primarily to manage resources, quality and the environment.

Management is, of course, a subject in its own right with training available worldwide and a vast literature (e.g. Reynolds *et al.*, 2003). An important training design issue is to distinguish, from the broad swathe of management studies, elements which relate directly to the management of residential and boarding settings. The key purpose is to manage a service that safeguards and promotes young people's well-being and developmental potential. A competent manager should demonstrate a leadership style that develops a culture of open and participatory management and practice, and ensures that staff are managed and supported to deliver a quality service. The main roles for this have been distinguished as follows:

- provide leadership and management of the residential task;
- manage a provision which safeguards and promotes the well-being of young people and enables them to reach their developmental potential;
- manage people;
- manage a quality service.

(TOPSS, 2003)

The complete model allows the identification of the elements of a quality service, all of which require management. Staff are concerned, directly or indirectly, with all the components and therefore the management of people is vital. The purpose of the system is to promote the well-being of the young people and to encourage them to realise their potential. To manage successfully all facets of a residential and boarding education and care establishment requires leadership of a high order together with a wide range of knowledge and skills, which can be identified by the model.

The supervisory management programme available under the UK government's EduCare programme identified the following sectors of management:

- team-work and relationships;
- yourself;
- people;
- activities;
- projects;
- resources;
- quality;
- information.

All of these criteria may be derived from the model although, instead of 'projects', the term 'change' is preferred. The management model may be annotated to show the main managerial aspect of each element, thereby providing guidelines for the entire management process (Figure 6.2). As an example, child protection is fundamental to the management of quality. The maintenance and development of the physical environment is mainly the concern of resource management. The monitoring and assessment of personal and social development clearly involves the staff team but also the management of data. If time is the fourth dimension in the model, management is the fifth dimension, for which the complete model provides a structure.

The basis for management in a residential or boarding environment at the house or group level is discussed in detail by Halliwell (1994). The four main themes for effectiveness are identified as:

1   Management and motivation.
2   Leadership.
3   Team building.
4   Organisation and time management.

Motivation is related to the clarity of structure and communication within the organisation, the working conditions, interpersonal relations, job satisfaction and the opportunity for responsibility, advancement and personal growth. Leadership styles vary but an effective leader must be both an executive, who can make decisions, and a developer, with trust in the team. The development of a team allows a greater variety of problems to be tackled in that a greater diversity of knowledge, skill and experience is deployed. Furthermore, team-working boosts morale, and recommendations are owned by the team as a whole and are therefore more likely to be implemented. Handy and Aitken (1986) suggest that, for a team, there is a growth cycle which follows the following stages:

- *forming*: acclimatisation;
- *storming*: a period of conflict while the aims are established;
- *norming*: settlement into an acceptable way of working;
- *performing*: the mature and productive phase.

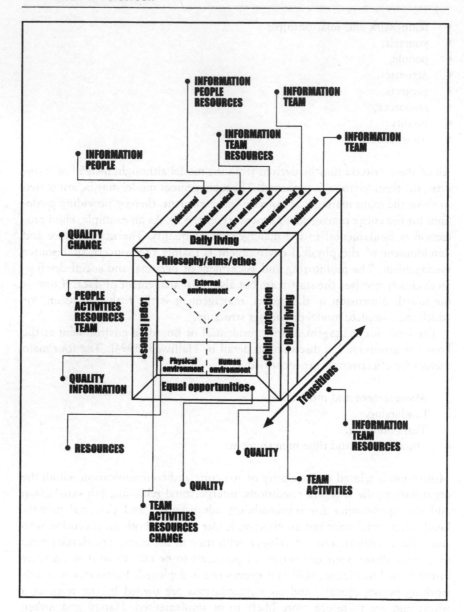

INFORMATION
PEOPLE
RESOURCES

INFORMATION
TEAM

INFORMATION
PEOPLE

INFORMATION
TEAM
RESOURCES

INFORMATION
TEAM

Educational   Health and medical   Care and welfare   Personal and social   Behavioural

QUALITY
CHANGE

Daily living

Philosophy/aims/ethos

External
environment

PEOPLE
ACTIVITIES
RESOURCES
TEAM

Legal issues

Child protection

Daily living

QUALITY
INFORMATION

Physical
environment   Human
environment

Transitions

Equal opportunities

RESOURCES

QUALITY

INFORMATION
TEAM
RESOURCES

QUALITY

TEAM
ACTIVITIES

TEAM
ACTIVITIES
RESOURCES
CHANGE

Figure 6.2 Model for management

Organisation and time management involves many of the aspects of residential living but particularly communication and line management. The art is to be available to colleagues and young people as appropriate while also making the best use of time.

For all staff at any level of management, complete familiarity is required with the basic structure of the establishment. This includes not only the fabric and the staff but the policies, procedures and records. A useful guide to these is produced in the Appendices of National Minimum Standards for Boarding Schools (2002e). Among the policies and documents are listed: staff handbook, bullying policy, child protection policy, discipline including punishments, complaints procedure, policies with regard to contemporary hazards, medical policy and protocols, health and safety policy, and policies directed at various emergencies. Among the records which need to be kept are those connected with child protection, major punishments, physical restraint, serious complaints, significant illnesses, accidents and injuries, parental permissions, risk assessments, fire and emergency precautions, and records of each young person. The establishment should also keep a running record of items which need to be monitored including: complaints, major punishments, physical restraint, risk assessments and medical factors such as medication, treatment and first aid and significant accidents.

Research and development

Apart from its role in course design and training, the main application of the model so far has been in research and development. Its initial use was at the first York Day (2001), attended by practitioners and researchers from all the main types of setting together with representatives from the relevant government departments. The purpose was to identify subjects which are common across the variety of types of setting and which require further research. For example, the factors which govern status in any group of young people are of interest throughout the entire field. As indicated in Chapter 2, there is strong evidence from all sectors of residence and boarding that there are shared values. Indeed, the commonly accepted list of such values itself provides a good example of transfer from residential care for adults to the care of young people. Unit capacity, group size and the peer group provide other examples of common concern which require further research.

Whether the research is generated internally or by external bodies, the model is equally applicable. However, particularly through its links to training, it is hoped that familiarity with the model will encourage more practitioner research (Fuller and Petch, 1995). Staff living and learning with the young people are obviously well placed to monitor and assess the activities of the young people in an unobtrusive manner (Webb et al., 2000). Indeed, action research (e.g. Stringer, 1999; Winter and Munn-Giddings, 2001) is seen increasingly as an important element of social research, and those who work with the young people on a daily basis are in a good position to adopt a wide range of measures to assess change (Milner and O'Byrne, 2002). The issues of participant observation and perhaps bias are likely to arise but these may be addressed, if necessary, with suitable support from the external environment. Staff can develop the habit of standing back so that things may be seen in perspective.

Apart from the potential research topics identified by the use of the model (Figure 6.3), many of the procedures result in the collection of data which form the basis for research programmes. The preview and review of each duty session, risk assessments of all types and monitoring of individuals and groups all provide examples. Indeed, diligent and sensitive monitoring and measured assessment followed by the careful recording of data and the production of reports is fundamental to both good practice and research (Burgess, 1984). Apart from the possibility of personal development and advancement for staff, such research is of particular utility in complementing materials collected for inspections. Since inspections last at the most for a few days, it is impossible for many aspects of the assessment to be anything other than superficial. If there are continuous records, these can supplement the work of the inspectors and enhance the inspection system.

Inspections provide only one instance of the potential impact of research, albeit one of perhaps immediate concern. Of greater long-term importance is the role which research results can play in the development of the setting to increase the possible benefits for young people in residence or boarding. If improvements are to be made, all aspects of the environment and life within it need to be under constant review. For the entire establishment, policies and procedures may require amendment while, for the individual, activities may need to be changed and care plans adjusted. Progress at all levels depends upon the enthusiasm, perception and diligence of staff. In residential and boarding education and care, research is highly dependent upon meticulous observation and the recording of what in themselves might appear to be minor events. The adoption of a research mindset not only gives the staff member a greater stake in the development of the establishment but also provides an added source of interest in the daily round.

An example of how such a procedure can relate directly to an everyday concern of compelling interest across the field is provided by internet monitoring. The potential dangers for young people of internet use have been discussed (Chapter 4) and at present there is an over-dependence upon filter and blocker-based technology for protection. These are not effective where communications are being attempted between individuals using images, email attachments, audio or video streams, or where messages are either being generated or read off-line. In these cases, to identify computer abuse requires specific monitoring products. Residential staff are particularly well placed to monitor approaches to protection so that an effective system may be developed and maintained for the benefit of all young people.

However, it is in the area of transfer from one sector or setting to another that the model suggests the greatest scope for research. Subjects such as length of stay, family links, values and developmental stages are all applicable throughout residential and boarding education and care, and all are known to be under

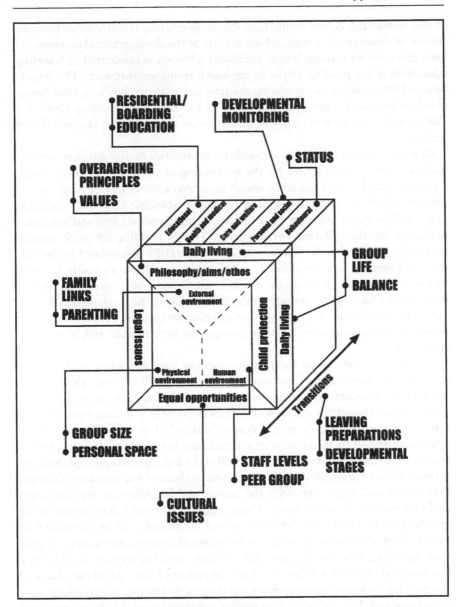

Figure 6.3 Model for research and development

scrutiny. Considerations of this type of issue are included in the evaluation of the *Children Act* (1989) (DoH, 2001).

Transfer between the different components of the model has already proved fruitful. Among the environmental components, the importance of group size and of various forms of therapeutic approach have been significant. Aims, one of the framework components, have shown interesting transfer value between several of the types of setting. Many aspects of the developmental components have potential for transfer but of particular relevance is residential or boarding education, a key product of the living and learning environment. The importance of after-care, a factor among the time components, has long been recognised in boarding schools, is the focus of the *Children (Leaving Care) Act* (2000), and is of growing interest and an issue for research in custodial care settings.

Current research which has crossed the boundaries of the different settings includes work on procedures for the monitoring of personal and social development, described in Chapter 5, which have been used in one or more special schools, children's homes, boarding schools, psychiatric units and custodial care establishments. Another issue under current examination is staffing ratios necessary for the different environments. This is building on work already undertaken by the Residential Forum (2002). The DfES is interested in the benefits of boarding and the different types of young people currently in other forms of residence who might be able to fit into mainstream boarding. Research is underway to develop methods of isolating the residential or boarding factor from what is a multivariate situation so that the benefits for young people of living away from home in groups may be identified and, if possible, enhanced.

Previous research set in forty-three boarding schools looked at the use of time, contact between staff and young people and activity centres. Duty time in the human environment is generally so occupied by activities and routines that a high proportion of the pastoral effort has to occur in non-duty time. Staffing ratios in boarding schools are, of course, relatively low and there were some interesting results in the context of contact time between the staff and boarders. In some schools, it was found that well under half the young people had any formal contact with staff during a week. An analysis of the interaction showed that most interactions were with the seniors and high-fliers or the miscreants and malcontents. In other words, those academically and behaviourally in the middle who, in a real sense fulfil the aims of the school, may be generally neglected. Work on activity centres, the locations of greatest interaction, showed that the dining area was of particular relevance. In other settings, similar work has revealed that the kitchen is often the centre of life. All these pieces of research have resulted in some change in the establishments, as procedures have been improved. In a custodial care setting, the initial work has been completed on the leaving procedure and ensuring that the monitoring system for personal and social development in custody is continued in a seamless fashion in the community.

As the model is used in residential and boarding practice, so ideas for research can be generated. The primary aim of such research should be the improvement of life and expectations for the young people but an important secondary aim is the further professional development of the staff. Research should not be seen as some esoteric university-based procedure but as a normal part of everyday life in the residential setting (Bullock *et al.*, 1998a).

Wider application

Following the various meetings and research seminars, the model has attracted interest beyond the immediate field of residential and boarding education and care for which it was developed. It has been demonstrated that the model is equally applicable to FE colleges or boarding schools with possibly several hundred residents, and children's homes with perhaps as few as four or five young people. Therefore, it cannot be considered scale-specific and, since residential or boarding education and care equates closely with good parenting, it is not surprising that the same model may be adapted for application in fostering, some aspects of adoption and day care, and periods of temporary residence in, for example, camps and activity centres. The components can be refashioned to the scale of the family and many of the techniques are applicable to young people living in families. While the environmental components will be on a considerably smaller scale in the case of the family, the framework components are directly applicable, particularly those concerning parental responsibility. The model has been presented in mainstream day schools and the framework and developmental components, in particular, are directly transferable. Since the model provides a summary of good living and learning practice, it is not unreasonable to conclude that its application may be wider than that of residential and boarding education and care.

Prospect

The basic structure has proved robust, but the model continues to be refined and developed both theoretically and in its application. As new and hybrid settings emerge, their requirements can offer scope for the further transfer of good practice. The employment of the model for fostering and family-based life requires a marked reduction in scale while its use for temporary residence requires a considerable foreshortening of the time and developmental components. The current intention of the DfES that all young people of a certain age should spend some time in camp indicates a general acceptance that there are benefits of some sort which accrue from living together, even temporarily, in groups away from home. It is hoped that the model can therefore be deployed to assist in an accurate and precise assessment of the benefits of residence and boarding.

References

Aguilera, D.C. (1994) *Crisis Intervention: Theory and Methodology* (7th edn). St Louis: Mosby.

Ainsworth, F. and Fulcher, L.C. (eds) (1981) *Group Care for Children*. London: Tavistock.

Allen, N. (1992) *Making Sense of the Children Act* (2nd edn). Harlow: Longman.

Anderson, E.W. (1978) *Assessment of Boarding*. Boarding Schools' Association Occasional Paper 4. London: Boarding Schools' Association.

Anderson, E.W. (1993) The Aims of Residential Education and Care. In Anderson, E.W. and Davison, A.J. (eds) *Applying the Children Act (1989) in Boarding and Residential Education*. London: David Fulton, pp. 26–46.

Anderson, E.W. (ed.) (1994a) *In Loco Parentis: Training Issues in Boarding and Residential Environments*. London: David Fulton.

Anderson, E.W. (1994b) Discipline and Control. In Anderson, E.W. (ed.) *In Loco Parentis: Training Issues in Boarding and Residential Environments*. London: David Fulton, pp. 69–83.

Anderson, E.W. and Davison, A.J. (eds) (1993) *Applying the Children Act (1989) in Boarding and Residential Education*. London: David Fulton.

Anderson, E.W. and King, C. (1994) The Residential Environment. In Anderson, E.W. (ed.) *In Loco Parentis: Training Issues in Boarding and Residential Environments*. London: David Fulton, pp. 188–197.

Anderson, E.W. and Morgan, A.L. (1987) *Provision for Children in Need of Boarding/Residential Education*. Report to the Boarding Schools' Association.

Association of National Specialist Colleges (2001 and 2002) *Directory*. Grimsby: The Association of National Specialist Colleges.

Atherton, J.S. (1989) Interpreting Residential Life Values in Practice. In Douglas, T. (ed.) *Residential Social Work*. London: Tavistock/Routledge.

Berridge, D. (1985) *Children's Homes*. Oxford: Blackwell.

Berry, J. (1975) *Daily Experience in Residential Life – A Study of Children and their Care-Givers*. London: Routledge & Kegan Paul.

Blatchford, P. (1998) *Social Life in School*. London: Falmer Press.

Blatchford, P. (2003) *The Class Size Debate: Is Small Better?* Maidenhead: Open University Press.

Blumenthal, G.J. (1985) *Development of Secure Units in Child Care*. Aldershot: Gower.

Blyth, E. and Milner, J. (1997) *Social Work with Children: The Educational Perspective*. Harlow: Longman.

Boyd, R. (1999) *Running a School Boarding House*. London: Boarding Schools' Association.

Brady, E. (1993) *Coping with Violent Behaviour: A Handbook for Social Work Staff*. Harlow: Longman.

Brandon, M., Schofield, G. and Trinder, L. (1998) *School Work with Children*. London: Macmillan.

Brayne, H. and Martin, G. (1999) *Law for Social Workers* (6th edn). London: Blackstone Press.

Brearley, P., Hall, F., Gutridge, P., Jones, G. and Roberts, G. (1980) *Admission to Residential Care*. London: Tavistock.

Brothers, J. and Hatch, S. (1971) *Residence and Student Life: A Sociological Inquiry into Residence in Higher Education*. London: Tavistock.

Brown, A. and Bourne, I. (1999) *The Social Work Supervisor*. Buckingham: Open University Press.

Brown, B. and Christie, M. (1981) *Social Learning Practice in Residential Child Care*. Oxford: Pergamon.

Brown, E., Bullock, R., Hobson, C. and Little, M. (1998) *Making Residential Care Work: Structure and Culture in Children's Homes*. Aldershot: Ashgate.

Bullock, R., Gouch, D. and Little, M. (1998a) *Children Going Home*. Aldershot: Ashgate.

Bullock, R., Gouch, D., Little, M. and Mount, K. (1998b) *Research in Practice*. Aldershot: Ashgate.

Bullock, R., Little, M., Ryan, M. and Tunnard, J. (1999) *Structure, Culture and Outcome: How to Improve Residential Services for Children*. Dartington: Dartington Social Research Unit.

Burgess, C. (1981) *In Care and Into Work*. London: Tavistock.

Burgess, R.G. (1984) *An Introduction to Field Research*. London: Routledge.

Burton, J. (1993) *The Handbook of Residential Care*. London: Routledge.

Burton, J. (1998) *Managing Residential Care*. London: Routledge.

Callow, M. (1993) Communication Need. In Anderson, E.W. and Davison, A.J. (eds) *Applying the Children Act (1989) in Boarding & Residential Environments*. London: David Fulton, pp. 121–139.

Callow, M. (1994) Relationships. In Anderson, E.W. (ed.) *In Loco Parentis: Training Issues in Boarding and Residential Environments*. London: David Fulton, pp. 84–105.

Casson, S.F. and Manning, B. (1997) *Total Quality in Child Protection: A Manager's Guide*. Lyme Regis: Russell House.

CCETSW (1978) *Good Enough Parenting*. London: Central Council for Education and Training in Social Work.

Chakrabarti, M. and Hill, M. (eds) (2000) *Residential Child Care – International Perspectives on Links with Families and Peers*. London: Jessica Kingsley.

Charterhouse Group (2001a) *A Living Learning Situation*. London: Charterhouse Group.

Charterhouse Group (2001b) *Standards for Therapeutic Community Childcare, Health and Education*. London: Charterhouse Group.

Children's Placement Finder (2004) London: CareandHealth.

Cigno, K. and Bourn, D. (eds) (1998) *Cognitive-behavioural Social Work in Practice*. Aldershot: Ashgate.

Clough, R. (2000) *The Practice of Residential Work*. Basingstoke: Macmillan.

Cole, T. (1986) *Residential Special Education*. Milton Keynes: Open University Press.

Coleman, J.C. and Hendry, L.B. (1999) *The Nature of Adolescence* (3rd edn). London: Routledge.

Coles, B. (2000) *Joined-up Youth Research Policy and Practice: A New Agenda for Change?* Leicester: Youth Work Press.

Colton, M., Sanders, R. and Williams, M. (2001) *An Introduction to Working with Children: A Guide for Social Workers*. Basingstoke: Palgrave.

Cooke, N.M. (1993) Is it Safe to Touch? In Anderson, E.W. and Davison, A.J. (eds) *Applying the Children Act (1989) in Boarding and Residential Education*. London: David Fulton, pp. 164–177.

Cooke, N.M. (1994) Special Issues: Sex, AIDS and Drugs. In Anderson, E.W. (ed.) *In Loco Parentis: Training Issues in Boarding and Residential Environments*. London: David Fulton, pp. 171–187.

Coulshed, V. and Mullender, A. (2001) *Management in Social Work* (2nd edn). Basingstoke: Palgrave.

Coulshed, V. and Orme, J. (1998) *Social Work Practice: An Introduction* (3rd edn). Basingstoke: Macmillan.

Courtioux, M., Davies Jones, H., Kalcher, J., Steinhauser, W., Tuggener, H. and Waaldijk, K. (1976) *The Social Pedagogue in Europe: Living with Others as a Profession*. Zurich: FICE (International Federation for Educative Communities).

Cowie, H. and Wallace, P. (2000) *Peer Support in Action*. London: Sage.

Crimmens, D. and Pitts, J. (eds) (2000) *Positive Residential Practice – Learning the Lessons of the 1990s*. Lyme Regis: Russell House.

Custodial Care National Training Organisation (2002) *Custodial Care Standards, NVQs and SVQs*. Newcastle-upon-Tyne: NTO.

Dartington Social Research Unit (2001) *Matching Needs and Services* (3rd edn). Dartington: Dartington Academic Press.

Davies, M. (ed.) (1997) Principle of Parental Involvement. In *The Blackwell Companion to Social Work*. Oxford: Blackwell.

Davis, L. (1982) *Residential Care: A Community Resource*. London: Heinemann Educational.

Davis, L. (1993) *Sex and the Social Worker* (new edn). London: Janus.

Davison, A. (1993) The Problem Decelerating Environment in Residential Group Care and Educational Settings. In Anderson, E.W. and Davison, A.J. (eds) *Applying the Children Act (1989) in Boarding and Residential Education*. London: David Fulton, pp. 95–120.

Department for Education (Project Director: Smith, P.) (1994) *Bullying: Don't Suffer in Silence*. London: HMSO.

Department for Education and Employment (Architects and Buildings Branch) (1997) *School Grounds: A Guide to Good Practice*. London: The Stationery Office.

Department for Education and Skills (2001a) *Special Educational Needs: Code of Practice*. Nottingham: DfES Publications.

Department for Education and Skills (2001b) *Access to Education for Children and Young People with Medical Needs*. Nottingham: DfES Publications.

Department of Health (1988) *Protecting Children: A Guide for Social Workers Undertaking a Comprehensive Assessment*. London: HMSO.

Department of Health. Project Team: Social Services Inspectorate in the North West and Social Services Departments of Cheshire, Lancashire, Liverpool, Salford, St Helens and Tameside (1989a) *Homes are for Living In*. London: HMSO.

Department of Health (1989b) *An Introduction to the Children Act (1989)*. London: HMSO.

Department of Health (1991a) *The Children Act 1989. Guidance and Regulations. Volume 4: Residential Care*. London: HMSO.

Department of Health (1991b) *The Children Act 1989. Guidance and Regulations. Volume 5: Independent Schools*. London: HMSO.

Department of Health (1991c) *The Children Act 1989. Guidance and Regulations. Volume 6: Children with Disabilities*. London: HMSO.

Department of Health (1991d) *The Children Act 1989. Guidance and Regulations. Volume 7: Guardians Ad Litem and other Court Related Issues*. London: HMSO.

Department of Health (1991e) *The Children Act 1989. The Welfare of Children in Boarding Schools. Practice Guide*. London: HMSO.

Department of Health (1993) *Guidance on Permissible Forms of Control in Children's Residential Care*. London: HMSO.

Department of Health (1998a) *Caring for Children Away from Home*. London: The Stationery Office.

Department of Health (1998b) *Quality Protects*. London: The Stationery Office.

Department of Health, Home Office and Department for Education and Employment (1999) *Working Together to Safeguard Children: A Guide to Inter-agency Working to Safeguard and Promote the Welfare of Children*. London: The Stationery Office.

Department of Health (2000a) *Assessing Children in Need and their Families: Practice Guidance*. London: The Stationery Office.

Department of Health (2000b) *Framework for the Assessment of Children in Need and their Families*. London: The Stationery Office.

Department of Health (2001) *The Children Act Now: Messages from Research*. London: The Stationery Office.

Department of Health (2002a) *Accommodation for Students under Eighteen by Further Education Colleges. National Minimum Standards*. London: The Stationery Office.

Department of Health (2002b) *Care Homes for Younger Adults and Adult Placements. National Minimum Standards*. London: The Stationery Office.

Department of Health (2002c) *Residential Special Schools. National Minimum Standards*. London: The Stationery Office.

Department of Health (2002d) *Children's Homes. National Minimum Standards*. London: The Stationery Office.

Department of Health (2002e) *Boarding Schools. National Minimum Standards*. London: The Stationery Office.

Department of Health and Social Security, Advisory Council on Child Care (1972) *Care and Treatment in a Planned Environment*. London: HMSO.

Doel, M. and Sawdon, C. (1999) *The Essential Group Worker*. London: Jessica Kingsley.

Douglas, T. (1977) *Groupwork Practice*. London: Tavistock.

Eggert, M. (1999) *Perfect Counselling – All You Need to Get it Right First Time*. London: Random House Business Books.

Farmer, E. and Pollock, S. (1998) *Sexually Abused and Abusing Children in Substitute Care*. Chichester: Wiley.

Faupel, A., Herrick, E. and Sharp, P. (1998) *Anger Management*. London: David Fulton.

Fawcett, M. (1996) *Learning Through Child Observation*. London: Jessica Kingsley.

Finch, J., Hill, P. and Clegg, C. (2000) *The Health Advisory Service: Standards for Child and Adolescent Mental Health Services*. Brighton: Pavilion.

Findlay, R. (2000) *International Schools: The Database*. Tilshead, Salisbury: International Schools Limited.

Fitzgerald, B. (1994) Meeting Children's Needs. In Anderson, E.W. (ed.) *In Loco Parentis: Training Issues in Boarding and Residential Environments*. London: David Fulton, pp. 106–124.

Franklin, B. (2002) *The New Handbook of Children's Rights*. London: Routledge.

Fuller, R. and Petch, A. (1995) *Practitioner Research*. Buckingham: Open University Press.

Gabbitas Educational Consultants (2003–2004) *Schools for Special Needs*. London: Kogan Page.

Gahagan, J. (1975) *Interpersonal and Group Behaviour*. London: Methuen.

Geddes, R. and Gutman, R. (1977) The Assessment of the Built-environment for Safety: Research and Practice. In Hinkle, L.E. and Loring, W.C. (eds) *The Effect of the Man-made Environment on Health and Behavior*. Atlanta: US Department of Health, Education and Welfare, pp. 143–195.

Gottesman, M. (1991) *Residential Child Care: An International Reader*. London: Whiting and Birch.

Green Paper (2003) *Every Child Matters*. Green Paper presented to Parliament by the Chief Secretary to the Treasury by Command of Her Majesty (September 2003). London: The Stationery Office.

Gupta, R.M. and Coxhead, P. (1990) *Intervention with Children*. London: Routledge.

Halliwell, T. (1994) Management. In Anderson, E.W. (ed.) *In Loco Parentis: Training Issues in Boarding and Residential Environments*. London: David Fulton, pp. 37–68.

Handy, C. and Aitken, R. (1986) *Understanding Schools as Organisations*. Harmondsworth: Penguin.

Hargie, O., Saunders, C. and Dickson, D. (1994) *Social Skills in Interpersonal Communication* (3rd edn). London: Routledge.

Harrington, R. (2001) Confidentiality. In Holgate, T. (ed.) *Good Practice in Boarding Schools*. London: Boarding Schools' Association, pp. 76–87.

Harris, R. and Timms, N. (1993) *Secure Accommodation in Child Care*. London: Routledge.

Hawkins, P. and Shohet, R. (2000) *Supervision in the Helping Professions* (2nd edn). Buckingham: Open University Press.

Health and Safety Executive Books (1993) *Health and Safety in Residential Care Homes*. London: Health and Safety Executive.

Health and Safety Executive Commission (1995) *Managing Health and Safety in Schools*. London: HMSO.

Hill, M. (ed.) (1999) *Effective Ways of Working with Children and their Families*. London: Jessica Kingsley.

Hills, D.W. and Child, C. (2000) *Leadership in Residential Child Care*. Chichester: Wiley.

Hoghughi, M. (1980) *Assessing Problem Children: Issues and Practice*. London: Burnett Books.

Holgate, T. (ed.) (2001) *Good Practice in Boarding Schools*. London: Boarding Schools' Association.

Holgate, T. and Morgan, R. (2000) *Developing the Gap Assistant's Role*. London: Boarding Schools' Association.

Hollin, C.R., Epps, K.J. and Kendrick, D.J. (1995) *Managing Behavioural Treatment*. London: Routledge.

Horwath, J. (ed.) (2001) *The Child's World*. London: Jessica Kingsley.

Horwarth, J. and Morrison, T. (1999) *Effective Staff Training in Social Care*. London: Routledge.

Hunt, E.E. and Sullivan, E.V. (1974) *Between Psychology and Education*. Toronto: The Dryden Press.

Hutchinson, S. (1993) Emotional and Developmental Welfare in the Light of the Children Act (1989). In Anderson, E.W. and Davison, A.J. (eds) *Applying the Children Act (1989) in Boarding & Residential Environments*. London: David Fulton, pp. 47–72.

Hutchinson, S. (1994) The Need for Self-awareness when Caring for Children. In Anderson, E.W. (ed.) *In Loco Parentis: Training Issues in Boarding and Residential Environments*. London: David Fulton, pp. 125–139.

Inman, S., Buck, M. and Burke, H. (1998) *Assessing Personal and Social Development: Measuring the Unmeasurable?* London: Falmer Press.

Investors in People UK (2000) *The Investors in People Standard*. London: Investors in People UK.

Irving, J., Munday, S. and Rowlands, A. (1993) *Pathways into Caring*. Cheltenham: Stanley Thornes.

Iwaniec, D. and Hill, M. (eds) (1999) *Child Welfare Policy and Practice*. London: Jessica Kingsley.

Jack, R. (ed.) (1998) *Residential versus Community Care*. Basingstoke: Macmillan.

Jackson, A. and Eve, A. (2002) *Hospice Information: Directory 2002*. London: Hospice Information.

Jacobs, M. (2000) *Swift to Hear* (2nd edn). London: SPCK.

Kahan, B. (1994) *Growing up in Groups*. London: HMSO.

Kellmer Pringle, M. (1975) *The Needs of Children*. London: Hutchinson.

Lambert, R. (1966) *The State and Boarding Education*. London: Methuen.

Lambert, R. (1975) *The Chance of a Lifetime? A Study of Boarding Education*. London: Weidenfeld & Nicolson.

Lambert, R., Bullock, R. and Millham, S. (1970) *A Manual to the Sociology of the School*. London: Weidenfeld & Nicolson.

Lennox, D. (1982) *Residential Group Therapy for Children*. London: Tavistock.

Lishman, J. (ed.) (1991) *Handbook of Theory for Practice Teachers in Social Work*. London: Jessica Kingsley.

Little, M. and Mount, K. (1999) *Prevention and Early Intervention with Children in Need*. Aldershot: Ashgate.

London Child Protection Committee (n.d.) *London Child Protection Procedures*. London: London Child Protection Committee.

Long, M. (2000) *Family Encyclopaedia of Medicine and Health*. London: Robinson.

McCormack, M. (1979) *Away from Home*. London: Constable.

McDerment, L. (ed.) (1988) *Stress-care*. Surbiton: Social Care Association.

Maier, H.W. (1987) *Developmental Care of Children and Youth*. New York: The Haworth Press.

Mallinson, I. and Thomas, G. (1984) *Learning from Experience*. Surbiton: Social Care Association.

Maslow, A. (1943) A Theory of Human Motivation. *Psychological Review* 50, pp. 370–396.

Megginson, D. and Whitaker, V. (1996) *Cultivating Self-development*. London: Institute of Personnel and Development.

Mickleburgh, S. (2001) Eating Disorders and Self-Esteem. In Holgate, T. (ed.) *Good Practice in Boarding Schools*. London: Boarding Schools' Association, pp. 195–208.

Millam, R. (1996) *Anti-discriminatory Practice*. London: Continuum.

Milner, J. and O'Byrne, P. (2002) *Assessment in Social Work* (2nd edn). Basingstoke: Palgrave Macmillan.

Mitchels, B. and Prince, A. (1992) *The Children Act and Medical Practice*. Bristol: Jordan & Son.

National Children's Bureau (1999) *Improving the Health of Children and Young People in Public Care*. London: National Children's Bureau.

National In-patient Child and Adolescent Psychiatry Study (1999) *Standards for Child and Adolescent Psychiatric In-Patient Services*. London: Royal College of Psychiatrists' Research Unit.

O'Hagan, K. (ed.) (2000) *Competence in Social Work Practice – A Practical Guide for Professionals*. London: Jessica Kingsley.

O'Quigley, A. (2000) *Listening to Children's Views*. York: Joseph Rowntree Foundation.

Payne, M. (2000) *Teamwork in Multiprofessional Care*. Basingstoke: Macmillan.

Pitts, J. (1999) *Working with Young Offenders* (2nd edn). Basingstoke: Macmillan.

Porteous, J.D. (1977) *Environment and Behaviour: Planning and Everyday Urban Life*. Reading, MA: Addison-Wesley.

Purser, C. (1998) *Health, Safety and Welfare of Pupils: The Responsibilities of the Governing Body*. Kingston upon Thames: Croner Publications.

Quality Network for In-patient CAMHS (2001) *Standards for Child and Adolescent Psychiatric In-patient Services*. London: QNIC.

Read, J.W. and Clements, L. (2001) *Disabled Children and the Law*. London: Jessica Kingsley.

Redl, F. and Wineman, D. (1952) *Controls from Within*. New York: The Free Press.

Residential Forum (2002) *Care Staff in Care Homes for Younger Adults*. Surbiton: Social Care Association.

Reynolds, J., Henderson, J., Seden, J., Charlesworth, J. and Bullman, A. (2003) *The Managing Care Reader*. London: Routledge.

Robinson, C. and Jackson, P. (1999) *Children's Hospices: A Lifeline for Families?* London: National Children's Bureau.

Robinson, D. (1993) The Dark Side of Boarding. In Anderson, E.W. and Davison, A.J. (eds) *Applying the Children Act (1989) in Boarding and Residential Environments*. London: David Fulton, pp. 186–204.

Robinson, D. (1994) What is Boarding? In Anderson, E.W. (ed.) *In Loco Parentis: Training Issues in Boarding and Residential Environments*. London: David Fulton, pp. 1–19.

Rose, J. (2002) *Working with Young People in Secure Accommodation*. Hove: Brunner-Routledge.

Rose, M. (1997) *Transforming Hate to Love*. London: Routledge.

Rutter, M., Tizard, J. and Whitmore, K. (1971) *Education, Health and Behaviour*. London: Longman.

Safe on the Streets Research Team (1999) London: The Children's Society.

Scottish Executive (1999) *Click Thinking: Personal Safety on the Internet*. London: The Stationery Office.

Scottish Office (1992) *Another Kind of Home: A Review of Residential Child Care*. Edinburgh: HMSO.

Sharp, S. and Smith, P.K. (eds) (1994) *Tackling Bullying in Your School: A Practical Handbook for Teachers*. London: Routledge.

Shepherd, P. (1997) *National Child Development Study*. Institute of Education, London: Centre for Longitudinal Studies.

Silverman, D. (1970) *The Theory of Organisations*. London: Heinemann.

Sinclair, I. and Gibbs, I. (1996) *Quality of Care in Children's Homes*. York: Social Work Research and Development Unit, University of York Working Series Paper B, No. 3.

Sinclair, I. and Gibbs, I. (1998) *Children's Homes: A Study in Diversity*. Chichester: Wiley.

Smith, T. (2000) *BMA Complete Family Health Guide*. London: Dorling Kindersley.

Soisson, R. (ed.) (1992) *Policymaking, Research and Staff Training in Residential Care*. Zurich: FICE.

Stabis (2003) *Parents' Guide to Maintained Boarding Schools*. London: Boarding Schools' Association.

Stanley, D. and Reed, J. (1999) *Opening up Care: Achieving Principled Practice in Health and Social Care Institutions*. London: Arnold.

Stanley, N., Manthorpe, J. and Penhale, B. (eds) (1999) *Institutional Abuse: Perspectives Across the Life Course*. London: Routledge.

Stock, B. (1991) *Health and Safety in Schools*. Kingston upon Thames: Croner Publications.

Stock, B. (1993) *Health and Safety in Schools* (2nd edn). Kingston upon Thames: Croner Publications.

Stringer, E.T. (1999) *Action Research* (2nd edn). Thousand Oaks, CA: Sage.

The Violence Against Children Study Group (1999) *Children, Child Abuse and Child Protection*. Chichester: Wiley.

Thompson, N. (1997) *Anti-discriminatory Practice* (2nd edn). London: Macmillan.

Thomson, A. (2002) *Critical Reasoning: A Practical Introduction* (2nd edn). London: Routledge.

Training Organisation for the Personal Social Services (2003) *National Occupational Standards for Managers in Residential Child Care*. Leeds: TOPSS England.

Trotter, C. (1999) *Working with Involuntary Clients*. London: Sage.

Utting, W., Baines, C., Stuart, M., Rowlands, J. and Vialva, R. (1997) *People Like Us: The Report of the Review of the Safeguards for Children Living Away from Home*. London: The Stationery Office.

Varma, V. (1997) *Troubles of Children and Adolescents*. London: Jessica Kingsley.

Wade, J. and Biehal, N. with Clayden, J. and Stein, M. (1998) *Going Missing*. Chichester: Wiley.

Wagner, G. (1988) *Residential Care: A Positive Choice*. London: HMSO.

Walmsley, J. (1969) *Neill & Summerhill*. Harmondsworth: Penguin.

Ward, H. (ed.) (1995) *Looking After Children: Research into Practice*. London: HMSO.

Webb, E.J., Campbell, D.T., Schwartz, R.D. and Sechrest, L. (2000) *Unobtrusive Measures* (revised edn). Thousand Oaks, CA: Sage.

Willow, C. (1996) *Children's Rights and Participation in Residential Care*. London: National Children's Bureau.

Winnicott, D.W. (1957) *The Child, the Family, and the Outside World*. Harmondsworth: Penguin.

Winter, R. and Munn-Giddings, C. (2001) *A Handbook for Action Research in Health and Social Care*. London: Routledge.

Index

Note: page numbers in *italics* refer to figures.